This is a compelling account of
a couple had to face after a str
researched, scholarly, yet movin

Professor Sir Charles George
former Chairman of the Stroke Association UK

❀

This book is scholarly yet tender and personal, fiercely honest
and immensely confronting. It records the impact of stroke
and dementia and 'extreme care' on life and personality and
relationship. It is full of insightful comment and information
that could enable readers and carers in similar circumstances
to negotiate challenges with deeper understanding or to assist
others to do so.

I found it to be a poignant, costly and compelling account
that has gathered up two particular lives in a search for new
meaning in a context of profound loss. It stands as a testimony
to their commitment, for all those who loved them and for any
who may be on a similar journey.

Margaret Fuller
Social Worker, former Clinical Services Manager
Anglicare Counselling, Wollongong, NSW, Australia

"Extreme Caring" is an honest, sensitive and beautifully expressed account of the experience of long term caring for a loved one.

This book will not only resonate with carers, but enlighten those around them in the practical and emotional issues they face, and then delve deeper still by exploring value and meaning in life, caring and relationships.

I would thoroughly recommend this book to carers searching to make sense of losses and fully appreciate the value and significance of the things that remain.

Karen Cotton
Admiral Nurse Clinical Lead
Solent NHS Trust, Southampton, Hampshire UK

There have been other volumes on the caring journey of life with a brain-damaged or demented family member. This is a fine one, but it is much more. The reflections of a trained and intelligent mind on the meaning of caring and of life seen through the lens of "extreme caring" are relevant to us all.

The book meets the critical question following a reading. Do I wish to press it on my friends? A resounding "Yes".

Professor Sir Robert Boyd
formerly Pro-Vice-Chancellor, University of London

EXTREME CARING
CARING
-
YOU HAVE TO
GO ON

a search for meaning in life
with stroke and dementia

STUART DONNAN

for Mike and Ali,
my best friends and supporters

Contents

1. **"Dear Beryl, I hear that you have been struck down"**   **1**

Spring 2000   1

Struck down   2

To the reader   3

2. **"Why did Beryl have the stroke?"**   **5**

Why?   5

Beryl's medical history   5

The occurrence of the stroke   7

Beryl's report of her own experiences leading up to the stroke   9

Who does a stroke affect?   11

The strange effects of strokes: evolution, anatomy, and
     physiology   12

3. **"I want to walk – I'm sure I can walk"**   **17**

The first twenty-four hours   17

The 'Mondrian moment'   18

The rehab unit: to walk or to talk?   20

A star speech therapist   22

Dysphasia and aphasia   24

Paralysis and weakness   25

A lot less conversation: frustration and negotiation   26

4. **"Do you know what I mean?"**   **29**

The struggle to understand her words   29

Other sorts of meaning   30

Meaning for whom?   31

Stories and narrative   33

5.   "Hello Beryl, what's it like to have a stroke?"   **35**

What's it like to have a stroke?   35
Insights from my own experiences   36
Stubborn or persistent?   37
Discussing feminist theology – too much for the brain?   39
What the window cleaner saw   40
Drugs, more drugs, and more side effects   41
Other written experiences of stroke sufferers   42

6.   "I can't read – that's the hardest thing for me"   **45**

Now I can't read books   45
School books   46
Poetry and psalms   47
Bookshelves and feminist heroines   49
Writing   50
Watching   51
Talking and reading together   52
Reading and joining in   55

7.   "They're all memories that I just keep in my mind"   **59**

Bad dreams and bad memories   59
To sleep, perchance   60
Bad judgement   61
Good memories   62
Remembered activities and people   63
Remembered abilities, and forgotten ones   64
Interests and options   67
They're all memories   69
Those blue remembered mountains   70

8.   Lost for words – reflections written in 2004   **73**

Carers and creative writing   73

Words fail me – and her, and us 73
Lost for words – me, her, us, everyone? 77

9. "I thought she might have dementia" **81**

Not the D word, please 81
Learning about mental health and mental illness 82
Getting lost 83
Keep C-A-L-M and carry on? 84
Assessment 85
A consumer's view of research 87
Mind, memories and meaning 88

10. "Do you understand what I'm saying?" **89**

What about this? 89
Dementia and dysphasia affect words differently 91
A few good words 92
Humour in dysphasia and dementia? 94
Wine nonstop 98
Frustration, confusion, insight and sadness 99
But still trying to converse 103
You're in charge 105

11. "I'm sorry I'm not coping." "Well you have to." **107**

I'm sorry I'm not coping 107
Burnout and meaning 109
Losing it completely 111
Day care 112
Respite and care 115
I am weary and I wish … 118
The unkindest cut 122
Relentless 124
Extreme caring 124

12. **"The people in that place had no idea of life,**
    the universe, or …"   **127**

    From day centres to care homes   127
    Fading – and the fading of the light   131
    Accepting help   132
    The worst thing   134
    Abandonment   135
    Conceding defeat   136
    Long term care   137
    Contented – or not?   142
    Extreme care   144
    Thinking about meaning   146

13. **Meaning in images**   **147**

    Rehabilitation   147
    Talking with pen and paper   148
    A room with a view   149
    Art and life   152
    Still life   152
    Landscapes live and painted, and everyday scenes   154
    Galleries and portraits   159
    Beryl's Life Story Book   163
    A room of one's own   164

14. **Meaning in music**   **167**

    All that is left for me is the music?   167
    Music and rehabilitation   168
    Music and memory   169
    Music visible   171
    Music lifts the heart   172
    Music lifts the words   175
    Music and meaning   177

Music and acceptance – maybe rueful 178
Harmony in music – and everywhere? 179
Silence more lovely than music? 181

15. Meaning in silence **183**

The inexpressible 183
The silence of watching 184
The silence of waiting 185
Silence and stillness, alone or together 188
What sort of meaning in silence? 190

16. The meaning is in the caring **193**

Caring in context 193
Beryl as a carer – what she cared about 194
Evolution and costly cooperation 199
Global ethics 202
Care ethics 204
Achievative or affiliative? 206
Duty and joy, love and trial 207
Imperfect or impotent caring 210
Caring, loss and death 213

17. You have to go on **217**

How long? 217
In our sixteenth year 218
I can't go on like this 218
Why do you have to go on? 219
She has to go on 220
We have to go on 221
Rage or consolation? 224

Acknowledgements **227**
Notes and Sources **229**

"Dear Beryl, I hear that you have been struck down"

Spring 2000

It was the first spring of the new millennium. Old friends from Hong Kong days were visiting, and we went for a weekend walk on the South Downs near our holiday home on the English Channel south of London. The weather was fine and warm, and our visitors were energetic.

First we walked though a wood with wide stretches of bluebells, then along a stream, then through a gate onto a hillside field of corn up to waist height. By this stage our visitors were well ahead, striding up the modest incline. Beryl, my wife, was some way behind; when she was small her father used to say that she was built for comfort, not for speed. I was trying to keep in the middle, which meant that when I arrived at the brow of the little hill I was quite alone. The air was still, the sky cloudless and bright, and I was amazed to see and hear a skylark overhead. It was like van Gogh's painting of the wheatfield without the crows and their possible menace.*

But then some shadow of menace did appear, as Beryl came into view red-faced and breathless and quite distressed. I knew she was not especially fit, but this seemed more of a problem than I expected. She slowly settled, and we eventually met up with our friends back at the car. The day resolved slowly and quietly.

Struck down

On Saturday 20th May 2000, several weeks after that spring day, Beryl collapsed while we were visiting our son and his family and friends. I caught her as she fell; three of us present were doctors and we realised what was happening. An ambulance took her to the local hospital emergency department and she was admitted to the acute stroke ward.

After a week or so, a card arrived from a friend in London; a cosmopolitan clergyman known for his forthright speaking.

---

* I did not, at the time, know of his *Wheatfield with a lark* or that he shot himself near that wheatfield.

Full details for all the numbered references in the rest of the book are given in the 'Notes and Sources' section at the end of this book. The web address www.donnan.eu/extreme has full references and web links to music and other sources, as well as all the illustrations in original colour.

"Dear Beryl," he wrote, "I hear that you have been struck down."

Our experiences that followed were so absorbing and distressing that it was a full ten years before I could bring myself to revisit the details of that walk in the woods in my memory and write them down like this.

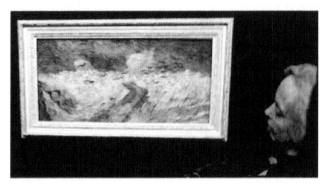

Beryl viewing van Gogh's *Wheatfield with crows* in Amsterdam from her wheelchair, thirteen years after her stroke

To the reader

I have written this book for those who wish to understand more about what it is like to live with a stroke and the subsequent illnesses and disabilities, especially disturbances of memory. It is also for those who are caring for, or have cared for, people with problems like these. It aims to acknowledge the challenges we face as carers as well as our varying success, and our frequent feelings of failure. In addition, the book describes how Beryl and I looked to find some sort of meaning in all the things that happened to us and around us.

I have separated into a second book* my philosophical and theological reflections about these illnesses, about living with and caring for them, and about looking for meaning. The separation is partly because of length, and partly because while some readers may be very concerned about those aspects, other readers may not be particularly interested.

---

* The companion book is *Faith When Words and Memory Fail: reflections on a spiritual life with stroke and dementia*; see Notes and Sources.

2

"Why did Beryl have the stroke?"

Why?

Shortly after the stroke happened, my aged mother asked me "Why did Beryl have the stroke?" It seemed to be a question more about meaning than about facts, but I am not sure, and my mother seemed satisfied when I answered in physical and medical terms.

Beryl's medical history

For nearly five years, Beryl had been under the care of very good local doctors in Manchester and then in London. She had complained of occasional short-lived palpitations, but various tests and heart tracings by the GPs had shown nothing of note. A few weeks after the cornfield episode, Beryl went to our GP in London feeling very unwell. For the first time, a heart tracing (an ECG) showed a real abnormality: atrial fibrillation, the name given to rapid contraction of the upper chambers of the heart which causes irregular contractions of the lower chambers of the heart, and thus an irregular pulse rate. The doctor prescribed digoxin, the standard treatment, and asked for an urgent scan at the local hospital of international repute to check for blood clots in her heart.

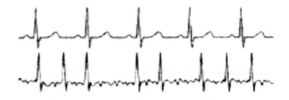

A normal regular heart rate tracing above an irregular heart rate tracing from atrial fibrillation

The GP whom Beryl consulted was working with me on a research project at the time. He spoke to me by telephone and mentioned that there had recently been discussions in some medical journals about whether drugs to slow the clotting of the blood might be used as standard treatment in such cases to prevent blood clots breaking off from the walls of the chambers of the heart. The GP decided to wait for the result of the urgent heart scan, and I concurred.

The occurrence of the stroke

About two weeks later, we went to stay with our son and his family in Southampton for the weekend. Beryl had not yet received an appointment for the urgent heart scan. That morning she was very slow in getting up and ready, which was unusual for her. We had a pleasant lunch in the garden of our son's house with the company including three doctors, a nurse and a radiographer. Towards the end of lunch she stood up, then mumbled something and began to fall. I caught her, and before we laid her down we all knew that she had suffered a stroke. Blood clots from her heart had, I presumed, broken off and blocked the blood supply to part of her brain.

An urgent ambulance took Beryl to the local hospital where the three doctors among us had all worked in the past. In the Accident & Emergency department, where I had been a consultant twenty years previously, the young doctor was concerned and helpful. However, she said that it was not clinically clear whether the stroke was due to a haemorrhage or a clot, and that over the weekend no brain scan was available to make that vital distinction. With the history, I thought that a clot was clearly the cause, but without the scan the doctor felt unable to give a clot-busting drug that, if indicated, might have minimised the effects of the stroke.

Beryl was taken to the acute stroke ward that seemed full of elderly women lying flat in bed. It was not a cheerful place, but Beryl was entirely unaware. We left her there and had a sleepless night; I was very absorbed with the idea, the desire, that she might not feel comfortless.

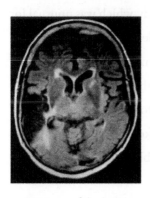

MRI scan of the head showing on the left a dark grey area of brain damage caused by a stroke

When the MRI scan was finally taken a few days later, it showed a large, dense, grey area of damage on the left side of Beryl's brain, in the middle between front and back, like that shown in the photograph. Being on the left side, it would be expected to have an impact on language as well as on movement.

The stress of the family then, and subsequently, was increased by questions about the control of Beryl's blood pressure over the years, as well as by the lack of investigations (and thus possibly treatment) at the acute stage on admission. In addition, I was somewhat distracted by the idea that the drug which she had been given to strengthen her heart beat, when the irregular heart beat was discovered, might in fact have caused the clot to break off. Even now, there is little research evidence about that specific point. The fact that the hospital had not managed to perform the heart scan when requested by the

GP, which may well have shown abnormalities leading to Beryl being given blood-thinning drugs precisely to prevent a stroke, was almost too painful to contemplate. But this was all in the year 2000, and the prevention, investigation and management of strokes are, we are led to believe, rather better organised in the NHS now than they were then; take, for example, the National Stroke Strategy of December 2007.[1]

Beryl's report of her own experiences leading up to the stroke

Beryl was interviewed five years after the stroke by a psychotherapist, who was also trained as a nurse.[2] The following are some verbatim extracts describing Beryl's memories of the time leading up to her admission to hospital. One of the major effects of Beryl's stroke was *dysphasia*; the disturbance of speech and language. I will give many more examples later, but the recorded interview illustrates it well.

> *About her heart irregularity in Manchester and then after coming to London in 1997:*
> I said to Stuart, "Oh, I feel really funny", and he just said, "Lie down and just...", you know, ... later on I didn't hear it again for a while, ... we went to London and we had to find doctors there ... and some of them, I think, didn't pay attention, you know, they

couldn't find anything wrong with me. But anyhow there was one woman, ... and I get a sort of tracing thing stuck round my middle, you know, for a whole day, and got that ... And every time they always said, "Well, there's no problem, there's no problem". And I would think oh well that's good, sort of thing!

But I think we'd been there for two years I think, in London ... I was very cross in my heart because I knew something was queer and funny; and sometimes I would wake up in the night and I knew it was beating and it was funny. And you know I thought, it took three or four hours before I could go to sleep and things like that, and at that time Stuart was working and so I didn't want to make a fuss. But anyhow over time there was one particular day and they only had appointments for people if they were really ... and this time I said to myself, I said, "Look, I am really sick, I feel horrible". And so I got a taxi or a bus or something and that particular chap there ... But actually he said, "I'm going to give you to the nurse to check it". And I was lying there and the nurse said, I'm sure she shouldn't have said this she said, "Wow! What have you been doing?" or laughing or something like that; and so I said, "Oh well I don't feel very well and so that's why...."

And then the doctor, he rang up three or four days later on and he said, "How do you feel?" And I said, "Oh, so much better!" and I was all chirpy and lovely... and we had these pills that I was having ...

About the occurrence of the stroke in May 2000:

... we were going to Southampton with my family there and we went on a train, you see, and I felt very well and I sat outside.

It was a lovely day with friends ... and suddenly... I didn't know what happened, suddenly it was just gone. It disappeared and I got... and I only saw one minute, I was sitting out in the garden, in their house, and I looked around and the only thing that I remember, they were all doctors, they were all coming around.

And the next thing, I didn't see till the next day when I had vagueness about anything... about anything had happened... But the next day I was in a ward ...

Who does a stroke affect?

A very helpful clinical neuropsychologist – a specialised counsellor – saw Beryl several times in the first few years after the stroke. She remarked rather pointedly, but on balance helpfully, "Doctors seem to think that strokes happen to brains – they don't, they happen to people."

Strokes affect people of all ages. High blood pressure, often with hardening of the arteries, is a common cause of stroke, and increasingly common with increasing age. Heartbeat irregularities, especially atrial fibrillation, are also a common cause, as in Beryl's case. Those irregularities can occur at younger ages. Beryl was sixty-two when the stroke happened, and several years younger when the heart irregularities began. Malformations of the blood vessels, including aneurysms (abnormal ballooning of the arteries), within the brain can also affect younger people; even children.

Details of how common stroke is in the UK, and a wealth of other useful information, are available from the Stroke Association.[3]

The strange effects of strokes: evolution, anatomy, and physiology

In quiet moments, or even in the heat of caring, it has occurred to me to wonder how and why the events that happened within my wife's body caused such devastating effects. Why the fibrillation? Why the left side of the brain? Why the damage to speech, and to reading and writing? Why the muscle weakness and its location? What is the 'meaning' of these things – why is the human body as it is?

Medical students learn interesting things about heart rate, for example that it can be regularly irregular or irregularly irregular. But one of the many remarkable things about the human body is that the heart rate is, overall, quite regular. Of course, a heart would not be very effective in any organism if the beating was not coordinated and at least moderately regular. Heart muscle cells are different from muscle cells in a limb, in that the heart muscle cells contract and relax spontaneously in their natural state. But a system has evolved to regulate and coordinate the beating of the individual cells. This system is located within the nerves of the heart, and is further regulated from the higher nervous system and the brain. If the coordination of the beating of the human heart fails, it is difficult to control or restore it with drugs. In the twenty-first century, we take so-called pacemakers for granted. They are a vital development in health care, and a reminder as to how delicate is the natural control system of the beating of the heart. Occasional or paroxysmal atrial fibrillation is much more common than used to be recognised. That problem had become permanent in Beryl, as in many other people, for no explicit reason; perhaps it related to stress on the muscle cells from higher blood pressure and lower oxygen supply than normal.

Beryl's stroke affected the left side of her brain, entirely by chance between left and right, it seems. The picture shows the most common arrangement (in 75% of people) of blood flow out of the heart in the main vessel; the aorta. The large arrow shows the direction of flow. The small arrow shows where the clot from Beryl's heart travelled. The common carotid arteries supply blood to the head, including the brain, on the left and right sides separately.

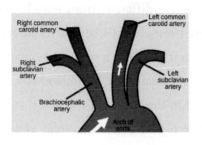

Sketch of the main blood vessels coming from the left side of the heart

What happens when clots go – again, presumably by chance – into the subclavian arteries that supply the shoulders and arms, or the external branches of the common carotid arteries that supply other parts of the head rather than the brain? The answer seems to be, first, that most of the clots that get into the circulation are very small, and second, that blood gets to most parts of the body from more than one artery. So a small obstruction can easily be bypassed by natural processes. The brain is more vulnerable in its blood supply, and particularly in the much shorter amount of time available, compared with other tissues, before serious damage is caused.

So, essentially by chance, the clot went into the left side of Beryl's brain. If it had been a much larger clot, she could have suffered what is often called a massive stroke, and died. If the clot had been smaller, its effects might have worn off fairly quickly. Instead, the consequences of Beryl's middle-sized stroke were weakness on the right side of her body, and a disturbance of speech and language, with other effects on intellect and memory. It was altogether life-changing; one might say life-shattering.

Neuroanatomy teaching as far back as my surgical training in the 1960s questioned the traditional focus on localisation of brain functions such as speech, and even of movement. But the affected side of the brain makes dramatic differences for patients such as Beryl, at least in the acute situation. Scientists in the twenty-first century still maintain "the brain's wrong-sidedness, or contralaterality, is one of life's great mysteries."[4] Movement and feeling on one side of the body are, to a large extent, controlled or focused in the opposite side of the brain. In practice, the effect of a stroke is usually very one-sided. Some people have a major problem with weakness or paralysis in the left side of the body, but no disturbances with speech and language.

Beryl's rapid and continued recovery from some, though far from all, of her problems is a demonstration of what has been called 'the plasticity of the brain'. In his excellent book *The Brain that Changes Itself,* Norman Doidge[5] describes how many losses and deficiencies in brain function are improved when different brain cells take over the functions of brain cells that have been destroyed. The amazing complexity of reading and writing is described in Maryanne Wolf's splendidly titled book *Proust and the Squid.*[6] The capacity for speech is hard-wired into the brain, and strokes and injuries interfere with the memory and understanding aspects of speech. But reading and writing are accomplishments learned new by every human individual, combining vision, memory and hand-eye coordination in separate parts of the brain. In some people, the learning of reading and writing does not develop well. In others, like Beryl, the learnt skills can be lost largely or completely when these combinations and pathways are interrupted.

So, the outward signs of the strokes affecting Beryl and others are the results of disturbing the amazingly complex anatomy and physiology, followed by further disturbance to social functions and the activities of daily life; especially those of communication.

3

"I want to walk – I'm sure I can walk"

The first twenty-four hours

On admission to hospital, Beryl was taken upstairs into a ward that to me seemed understaffed, and looked rather untidy. The ward was mostly full of little old ladies who were stroke patients, so it was not the most inspiring place. In the bed opposite Beryl there was a grey-haired woman, larger than the rest, lying there looking rather 'gaga' – that was the unpleasant and very unprofessional word that I am embarrassed to say came to mind. She had a tube in her nose, and was connected to various wires and other tubes. I was, understandably, rather depressed by all this.

When I saw Beryl the next morning she looked at me, then down at her right leg, then she made a little wiggling movement with her toes. And she said her first word: *Chuffed.* I was chuffed too, as recovery from the paralysis was beginning quickly. Later in the day, after more rest, the second word she said to me was *Organise!* We were staying with our son for the weekend when Beryl was admitted to hospital. We were living and working in London, while normally weekending in Rustington on the south coast. Beryl's old self was clearly functioning to some level, underneath all the problems of loss of movement and speech. *Organise* was just the word she would have used, and what was both appropriate and necessary if I was to be able to juggle work and hospital visits together with caring for two properties.

The next day our son visited by himself. As he was leaving, the woman in the bed opposite – whom I had ungraciously, as well as unprofessionally, labelled very negatively in my mind – sat up and said to our son, "Is that your mum? She's looking better." When I had first seen her she had, in fact, been lying there listening to music with headphones in her ears. She did have a tube in her nose because of a problem with swallowing. For me this was a very important reminder about not labelling, and about not judging by superficial appearances in environments like this.

The 'Mondrian moment'

A few days later, Beryl was moved to a side ward as she slowly recovered. Words were very restricted and mostly inaccurate. What names and numbers meant were anybody's guess. We were all grappling with a quite new experience of being inarticulate.

The metal sash windows of the side ward had secondary double-glazed windows that opened horizontally. The left side of the photograph below is of a window in a similar ward where she spent Christmas 2014, showing the houses and sky outside.

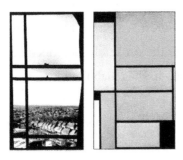

Hospital window on the left

Tableau I by Mondrian (1921) on the right; the dark spaces are red or blue or yellow in the original

When I came into the room, Beryl looked at me and then at the window before speaking one word: *Mondrian*. I was as encouraged as I was astonished. Despite the obvious damage to parts of her brain, some parts seemed to be still working very adequately, and she wanted to communicate her observations and thoughts to me. She remembered our visits to art galleries in Amsterdam, and our interest in Piet Mondrian as much as Van Gogh and the older masters. And this observation was based on the lines of the window panes without any of the colours that, although often in small sections, were fundamental to Mondrian's shapes and spaces. The perceptiveness of Beryl's memory in making the comparison is clear. This Mondrian moment was an important part of the beginning of her rehabilitation, and of our encouragement and rehabilitation together.

The rehab unit: to walk or to talk?

After two weeks Beryl was transferred to a rehabilitation unit on the edge of the New Forest in Hampshire. In the recorded interview, five years after the stroke, she described her recollections of the first few weeks in the rehabilitation unit.

> People were always popping out and going ... and then the other thing, I used to always see these little rabbits, when it was dark and I could watch them all and the place had horses, you know. I got so many cards and people – so many people – it was only later on when I thought it was really puzzling, so many people around me, you know, from a long way away, Norwich and other places, giving beautiful, lovely pictures, or presents and things like that ... But I thought it was very strange that everybody was making such a beautiful fuss, and one thing, all these blooms ... A few times, I noticed a few people who were much worse than I am and I found that was quite amazing.

It was a quiet, peaceful unit, as pleasant as such a place could be. In the first week or two, Beryl had more cards and flowers (the 'blooms' she referred to) than all the rest of the unit. Some of the severely disabled people were admitted for a short time for 'respite'; a word that I would become familiar with later on.

And then right near, with me, there was one lady who was all nursing [care], but she talked non-stop about everything. And I said, you know, I'll talk and she was talking so I talk, talk, talked and do all sorts of ….

After a while I said to somebody, that was Stuart I suppose, I said, "Look, I can't … I'm fed up with this sitting. I want to walk, I'm sure I can walk". And I think Stuart said, "Well have a go", … or something like that, and I felt I wasn't doing very well, and suddenly all these nurses raced round and said, "No, no, no, no! You don't want to that, you're not allowed to do that"! And I thought, oh-oh, and there was one nurse [*actually a physiotherapist*] and after a while she said, "Well, actually, you know, I've watched you for a while, you know, I think you could do it by now"… And I was so slow, she said, "Why do you moan, worrying all the time, just smile and …!" And after a time, I said, yes, after a while I found it so much better; and over time I was getting better and better with my walking around

A few days later on, this other woman who could talk non-stop – she was very amazed. She said, "Well if you can do it, I can do it!". … And I must say she tried very hard, but on the whole she was different to me and at the time I had no idea what the difference was. Because she said, "I need to work." In my mind I

21

was saying, "You're not going to be able to work like that". That was my idea. But I had these ideas myself about other people, all the time I was working things out.

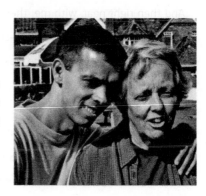

Beryl with our son Mike
on an outing from the
rehabilitation unit

So, after observing the other woman in the unit who could talk but not walk, Beryl, whose words were still very jumbled, began to work hard at walking. The physiotherapist encouraged her to try going up and down a few steps, because our house by the sea had three storeys. After a week or two, I was able to take Beryl home for a few hours with the help of friends. She came in the front door, hurried to the stairs, and walked up quickly to her favourite view of the sea. She came home to stay within another week or two.

A star speech therapist

In the rehabilitation unit, assistants came from the speech and language therapy section with flash cards to try to help Beryl get her words out. She was unable to name animals, for example. Overall, she was not at all impressed with the system.

When Beryl was able to return home, we were fortunate in that a member of the local award-winning community stroke team came to take on Beryl's speech and language therapy. She was as acutely perceptive as she was personable.

> I said to this woman, and she listened and I talked so much about I can't see any cats and dogs and all that silly business ... and then this lady said "Well, all right, we'll throw all that out of the way in the dustbin". And then she said, "We'll talk about things you like to talk about", and I think for a long couple of years after that I got so involved in talking with this lady. I want to go to Australia, and all sorts of things ... and after a while I got better and better

Very quickly, the therapist understood that Beryl wanted to talk about feminist issues and world development and justice, and about travel and about Australia. The therapist became as much a friend as was possible in the circumstances. She is one of a number of people whom we have come across who behaves in a way which affirms that there is much more to life than material concerns.

An occupational therapist also came occasionally for about a year. But there was a limited amount that she had to offer that Beryl could cope with.

Beryl said in the interview:

that occupational thing, I found it very, very boring! ... but she was a lovely gentleman ... lady I mean

The therapist showed her how she could dry the dishes with one hand, laying the teacloth on the bench, putting the cup or plate on it, and then wiping it with one hand. Beryl wanted to do the ironing; she had always enjoyed that. She managed some progress there, and helped a little for several years. Although I was uneasy, she never burnt herself.

Dysphasia and aphasia

Beryl's speech slowly improved, but she never recovered her fluency. The plasticity of the brain meant that the function of speaking, which was quite localised (though not completely), could be partly recovered by neighbouring parts of the brain. Good words, complex words, were sometimes there but not often.

My son, my daughter and I went to three different medical schools over a period of thirty years and more. Some things we learnt were very different, but some things changed very little, and that applied to many neurological problems. So we all discovered quickly that aphasia (loss of speech and language) and dysphasia (speech and language difficulties) were very different at home compared with the hospital bedside; one obvious difference was that, at home, you could not walk away to the next patient or to coffee. The nominal aphasia – the inability to say the name of an object such as a pen – that affected Beryl is really quite extraordinary, and quite interesting if you are standing at the end of a hospital bed. When you are trying to have an on-going personal conversation with the person, it is interesting but in a very different sort of way.

Reading has been a different matter. Reading for Beryl, and for everyone, is not hard-wired or built into the brain in the way speaking is, and she lost the ability to read. It has only even been the occasional individual word which registered correctly and which she could 'read'; that is, speak out loud.

Paralysis and weakness

The strength and function of Beryl's right leg recovered within a few weeks. But her right arm and hand lost their fine movements, and this never recovered. This loss meant that writing was impossible, except for the occasional word and printed signature during the first few years. I think the loss of writing has been in something of a negative feedback loop with the speech and reading. There has been no reinforcement or encouragement from one function to the other. And losing the dominant hand has lead to problems with the activities of daily living, such as using a toothbrush, with complex tasks around the house and driving our car becoming quite impossible.

A lot less conversation: frustration and negotiation

One of the early pieces of advice we had from the speech and language therapist was how stroke sufferers often lost some of their inhibitions, and how this could make negotiation difficult. On the one hand, I said that Beryl had never been particularly inhibited about saying what she thought. On the other hand, it did become enormously frustrating for both of us when discussing even simple matters, like choosing television programmes to watch, where it frequently became unclear what a *Yes* or a *No* meant. It could often mean the opposite, and could change upon repetition. *Open* and *Shut* had become of similarly unclear meaning.

I can remember literally banging my head on the wall, or on the patio windows, in the frustration of unsuccessfully trying my hardest to understand what she wanted, and to do it. I also remember the poignancy of feeling that Beryl, as a devotee of Virginia Woolf, was often speaking as if in a stream of consciousness, but a damaged or diverted one.

It became apparent that frustration implied insight. Beryl was aware of what she wanted to say or do, and also aware that it would not come out right. We tried technical assistance, for example special predictive word programmes on our computer, but they were quite beyond her capacity. We visited specialist agencies, but the main result of one visit was that Beryl declared her dislike of being with people who were disabled. We met several people whose dysphasia was much worse than Beryl's.

But another aspect of this speech and language problem, according to the therapist, is that people with dysphasia do not tell lies; there is no capacity for circumlocution. But, as with loss of inhibition, I did not think that this would be an issue with Beryl. For better or for worse, she had a reputation for being honest, often disarmingly so, and that remained an often-noted characteristic.

In our situations we usually coped, but it could be challenging in public. On one memorable occasion, we were buying window blinds in a department store. We had a loud and confused discussion about colours and designs, and the rather haughty staff member seemed to look down her nose (which was considerably elevated above our heads) at our behaviour. But we were not squabbling; I was simply trying to clarify just what Beryl preferred so that we could buy it.

I can understand that in regular interactions between adults, whether colleagues or couples, there is a distinction between clarification and negotiation. In clarification, the aim is to make clear what people's preferences or choices are. There may be no differences to settle, which is what negotiation traditionally involves. When Beryl's speech and language therapist brought up the topic that she called 'negotiation', she was aware of the special problem that we, and others like us, have had. In practice, the helper or carer – whoever is in discussion with the person with dysphasia – has great trouble knowing whether the task is to clarify or address differences. For me, the primary challenge was always to clarify. Negotiation, in the sense of settling differences, rarely arose. Perhaps this was partly due to our way of rubbing along with each other before the stroke. Awareness of this distinction may help, but that awareness does not seem to me to make the way forward any easier.

4

"Do you know what I mean?"

The struggle to understand her words

From the day Beryl suffered the stroke in 2000, we all began a struggle to comprehend what she was saying, and what she meant by what she said.

She frequently said, "Do you understand what I'm saying?" The honest answer, more often than not, was "Maybe". There are numerous examples in later chapters.

There seems something ironic in the fact that, as she was beginning to get her language back, one of the phrases Beryl would often repeat as a sort of stop-gap was *Over time*. Things did improve over time, that's for sure, but as time continued to pass, deterioration set in for other reasons, including us all simply getting older.

As the months and years advanced, so my struggle – our struggle – progressed to looking for broader meanings. This was not only with respect to health and illness, but also relating to life, the universe and everything.

Other sorts of meaning

I have already said that my mother's question "Why did Beryl have the stroke?" seemed to be a question about meaning, not just about facts. Some years later, good friends expressed their own questions about why such things had happened to us. I responded that I had never asked that sort of question. I was not, and am not, aware of or concerned about being singled out for special treatment, either bad or good. But I do have questions about why the world is as it is.

I also need to acknowledge that, not long ago, someone who was familiar with Beryl's progressing problems exclaimed, "Bloody God!" That reminded me of Francis Spufford's interesting book *Unapologetic*[7] where he makes something of a theme of similar words from Samuel Beckett's play *Endgame*[8] describing the strange situation where people are dissatisfied with a God whom they do not think exists. I have written my own theological and philosophical reflections on our experiences in the separate book *Faith when words and memory fail.*[9]

I will, quite consciously and deliberately, slip throughout this book between widely different meanings of the word *meaning*. These will include such notions as interpretation, translation, content, communication and, in contrast, purpose, value, significance, import, implication, relevance, or cause.

Meaning can be, as Terry Eagleton[10] says, what it all adds up to in life; perhaps, I think, the totality, the big picture. But he goes on to say that *meaning* can be what it all boils down to in life, which I think may be a different perspective on the big picture. Often, I am simply asking why various things happen or happened, and there is no need to force the actual word *meaning* into the question if it does not fit naturally.

Over the millennia, there have been innumerable discussions and pronouncements about the meaning of life. In the twentieth century, from existentialist philosophers to sociologists, such questions were raised about the meaning of life, or the lack of meaning in life. There is no need to pursue the topic from those perspectives here. But I saw recently a newspaper report of a conversation that the Dalai Lama had with a young waitress who spontaneously asked him what was the meaning of life.[11] He said that the answer was easy, namely happiness. But he added that the hard question, which all human beings must try to answer, was what produces happiness: money or accomplishment, or friends, or compassion and a good heart?

Meaning for whom?

These questions about meaning apply to me and to family members, to friends and acquaintances, but also, of course, to

Beryl herself. I have needed, in day-to-day life as well as in this book, to distinguish her from me, and also to do my best to ensure that she is included.

This book was originally going to be 'our' book, with me writing and then me reading each part to her for input and comment. But her disabilities advanced to the extent that this became impossible. My estimation of meaning for her thus was based on her recent and past demeanour, and on her comments from the past both distant and more recent being noted down by me, not by her. Fortunately, this can be supplemented by a variety of academic papers, sermons and journals she wrote in the past, before the stroke. Of particular value and interest is the lengthy recorded interview five years after the stroke, from which I have already quoted.

In our sort of situation, meaning, especially in terms of value, may often be ascribed or suggested by an onlooker, professional or otherwise. So sometimes, a third party is needed to evaluate, and validate, the thoughts and feelings of both the client/patient/sufferer, as well as the carer.

Rather more than the first half of this book describes the life we have led, Beryl's experiences and mine with her. The aim is, amongst other things, to show the complexities and challenges of her life, and to demonstrate how well she coped. The last four major chapters of the book are rather different. I will reflect more specifically on the aspects of our experience that have seemed to offer meaning to Beryl, and also to me. I need to mention, briefly, what I have not addressed directly in those chapters. Talking with friends about books in general, and about writing and music, I realise that, for me, it is largely the thinking and the talking that makes life worthwhile. No doubt this is partly a reflection of the limits on conversation that have been imposed on us by Beryl's illnesses. But it is more than that; it is the *search* for meaning which, to a large extent, has given my life meaning. Eagleton's book pointed that out quite clearly, but I have come to realise that I have been living out that fact. When I first wrote those words for myself, not much more than a year ago, I added "The rest is duty." I am not sure that I still think that. Certainly, I think that the second section of this book describes experiences and ideas that we have had and shared, and which have contributed to meaning in our lives, and lifted us, for a time at least, out of the mundane and away from the duty.

Stories and narrative

This book combines stories about our lives with reflections, and with some theoretical ideas. It is agreed, among many disciplines in the humanities, that we rely on narrative to make sense of our lives and to reassure ourselves that our lives are not pointless; that they have meaning. We make – indeed, even make up – our own stories about ourselves from our experiences and memories. Sometimes, the narrative of a person's life does become meaningless; unintelligible, even to his or her self. Physical and mental health problems are major causes of the meaningless that may develop.[12]

I am aware that I tell a lot of stories, and also frequently refer to poetry and to fiction. Jennie Erdal trained in philosophy, but as a journalist and a novelist she describes her agreement with Henry James's view: philosophy is a voice unsuited to reflecting the actuality of people's lives (I might add that the same often applies to theology). Erdal herself considers that some things, not least what it is that makes us human, can never be adequately expressed in conventional philosophical prose. She writes that reading novels brought her to feel that fiction was where truth was to be discovered.[13]

Thus, my struggle is to put several narratives, some in times of good health and some in times of ill-health, side by side with reflections on poems and novels and television. And to reach for meaning, perhaps, in the intersections. This is our on-going biography, one of the questions always being, "Who gets to decide on meaning?"

5

"Hello Beryl, what's it like to have a stroke?"

What's it like to have a stroke?

Less than a year after the stroke, we attended a wedding where we sat at the back of the church with our very small grandchildren. An acquaintance of many years sat down immediately in front of us. He turned around and said, in a loud voice, "Oh hello Beryl, what's it like to have a stroke?" We were rather taken aback, and Beryl was not able to respond at all. I mumbled something or other.

But it was not an unreasonable question. We have tried over the years to have some appreciation of Beryl's experiences, often indirectly because she has been mostly unable to articulate them.

About eighteen months after Beryl's stroke, we visited my very elderly mother in Australia for the first time since the stroke took place. She said to me afterwards, having observed Beryl's physical disabilities and her major difficulties with speech and language, "It's like a living death." The remark was not meant unkindly; rather, it was said with great sympathy. It was one observer's view of what it seemed like to have a stroke.

Insights from my own experiences

One of my clear memories from my first job as a junior hospital doctor was of helping care for an elderly man who was a stroke patient. On admission, he was semiconscious and his adult son, who was rather older than I was, asked me how he was doing. I remember saying, "Not too bad," mainly because I had no idea at that early stage how he was doing. The son retorted, "Not too good either!" I was sufficiently self-aware to feel somewhat chastened, and to realise that I was on a long learning curve. How could I know what it was like for the patient or for the family?

But I also recall, from time to time, an experience while working in the surgical unit at a London teaching hospital in the early 1970s. We had one small child at home, and family finances were very stretched. So, I jumped at the chance of being a research subject for colleagues in the internal medicine research group studying small bowel function, with compensation of £5. I had to swallow a large three-bore tube, and was given a small bottle of local anaesthetic for my mouth and throat to make the swallowing easier. I gargled and then swallowed the liquid. It seemed, without pausing to think about sensory nerve supply, the reasonable thing to do to ease the way down. But, of course, I was not supposed to swallow. I just did not pay attention to the instructions, or to what I was doing.

Over the next hour or two, as my body absorbed the large dose of local anaesthetic, I became increasingly weak in my limbs, and very conscious of the effort of breathing. I could think fairly clearly, and managed to get out the slurred words asking for the resuscitation trolley to be kept close by the bed. We agreed to go ahead with the research study since I would be on the bed for several hours anyway. The effects wore off after a few hours, and I was driven home with £5 in my pocket.

I remember discussing the experience with Beryl in bed at home that night, although I did not want to alarm her. It gave me some unasked-for insights into paralysis, and into being able to think but not communicate.

Stubborn or persistent?

Beryl's father was almost completely blinded in an accident when she was seven. As I got to know the family much later, he had a reputation for being stubborn. He persisted in trying to do many things at the limits of his capability. He continued building houses and walking on rafters in the incomplete roofs.

Beryl has been very stubborn in her attempts to recover and to continue with life after her stroke. I do not find that 'stubborn' is a bad word. She and her father both demonstrated admirable persistence and perseverance. In both cases, it has not always been without complication. Shortly after we were married, Beryl's father, with his very restricted vision, fell through the rafters on a house that he was building. He recovered, but was more restricted in his activities after the fall.

Beryl became able to look after herself at home while I worked a few days each week during the first few years after the stroke, but she needed help with many aspects of daily living. She was even able to walk to the local shops by herself with a shopping trolley. Between her and the staff who knew her, they managed to work out what she wanted, and to sort out the cash for payment.

But she was stubborn about some things that, for whatever reason, she did not think were a good use of my time and energy. Up to the time we had to abandon living in central London because of Beryl's stroke, I was the chair of the trustees of the Borough Market near London Bridge. One evening, about six months after the stroke, I had a meeting at the Borough Market, and when I returned to our apartment, she was not there. I anxiously enquired of friends nearby, and had visions of her lost, or worse, by accident or by design. Running out of ideas, I eventually telephoned our house in Rustington on the south coast. To my utter astonishment, which overshadowed my relief, Beryl answered the telephone. With her dysphasia she had managed to get from our apartment to London Bridge Station, get on and then off the correct train, get home in a taxi (it was too far to walk) and get into our house. To this day, I cannot quite understand how she achieved all that. But she was driven by her determination, albeit a determination partly based on disapproval of how I was spending my time and energy in London.

Discussing feminist theology – too much for the brain?

A year after the stroke, we were visited by old friends who had not seen the thesis that Beryl had completed about four years previously. It was for an MA in Theology with Feminist Studies, discussing "women-church" related to authority; quite a technical subject. Our friends read the thesis and discussed it with Beryl the next day. I was uncertain about the

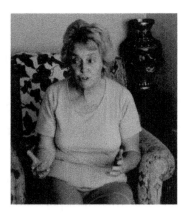

Beryl in 2001 in animated, if dysphasic, discussion of her writing

whole activity, but Beryl seemed capable of looking at her thesis and remembering some of what she had thought and written, and providing some sort of answers to their questions. This was despite her dysphasia, and what I think of as her *acquired dyslexia*; her inability to read out anything more than the occasional written word, and not always getting that right.

Our friends left the next morning. Later that day, Beryl telephoned me at my part-time work; it is hard to remember now that she was then able to use the phone. She reported having woken up on the floor some time in the afternoon. She had collapsed but did not know anything more about it.

What the window cleaner saw

Beryl collapsed at home several more times, with the circumstances not very clear. I was not there, and she seemed unhurt with no after effects.

One day, however, she collapsed in the living room while the window cleaner was on our balcony. He was a very pleasant chap, and it turned out that he had worked as a nurse. He took the initiative and let himself into the house. He called the ambulance, and Beryl was transported to the local hospital where she was admitted. The hospital then called me.

The problem was eventually diagnosed during her hospital admission as epilepsy. This was caused by scar tissue in the brain following the stroke, and apparently occurs in 5% of people within the first year after a stroke.[14]

Drugs, more drugs, and more side effects

Beryl was already taking warfarin and other tablets to reduce her risk of further stroke. It took six months from her hospital admission following the seizure to get the epilepsy medication right. Many of the drugs that were tried really slowed her down in both physical and mental activity. Even with the final choice, which was the least bad in terms of side effects, she became – and would remain – flat in comparison with her situation at one year, before the fits. This flatness persisted for a whole five years, until I persuaded the doctors to stop the medication.

It also took three or four changes to find blood pressure tablets that did not upset her. A well-known side effect of one of the drugs was to make the patient have a dry cough. Beryl was prescribed that drug and the dry cough appeared. She was able to sleep despite the cough, but I could not sleep at all. I was completely exhausted and I could not look after her, so we had to change the tablet for that reason. The side effect was thus in me, not in Beryl. This is not a traditional sort of side effect, but it may be more common than realised, because drug companies and doctors do not always take into account the big picture. In therapeutic situations like ours, the subject is more than the 'patient' being given the medication. Everyone involved in health care needs to understand the broad spectrum within which drug side effects may fall.

Other written experiences of stroke sufferers

Beryl was scarcely able to answer, for herself, the question about what it was like to have a stroke. She had brief contact with the excellent organisation called *Connect: the communication disability network* in south London,[15] whose publications include stories from stroke sufferers. I especially remember one young mother's story of coming home from hospital to her young children. They accepted her and her altered speech. Her small daughter introduced her to a school friend by saying, "This is my mum – she talks funny."

There are several books published by people who have recovered from a stroke sufficiently to resume fluent communication. By the nature of the illness, people whose stroke affected the other side of the brain from that affected in Beryl's stroke are the ones who retain speech and often the ability to write. But Jill Bolte Taylor, who suffered from a stroke as severe, and on the same side (the left), as Beryl's, was able, after eight years, to record her experiences in the excellent book *My Stroke of Insight*.[16] The journalist Robert McCrum suffered a massive stroke, but within three years published *My Year Off: Rediscovering Life After a Stroke*.[17] Tom Balchin suffered a major stroke affecting the right side of his brain as an undergraduate. After slowly returning to his studies, he published, fourteen years after the stroke, not an autobiography but rather a manual for others that he called *The Successful Stroke Survivor*.[18]

In Beryl's situation, we have my thoughts recorded here, but fortunately the recorded interview gives her a chance to produce some parts of an autobiography. Here she offers an opinion in 2005 about how people in general relate to strokes, or to people with strokes.

> I suppose I'm much more aware about other people who have no idea about anything medical of any sort, ... in the earliest days when he was, Stuart was, a surgeon ... all the other people would talk to me about that sort of work ... certain things like surgeons, a lot of the things are quite interesting for other people but honestly though nobody cares a hoot about strokes, really it's just one of those... no-one ...

6

"I can't read – that's the hardest thing for me"

Now I can't read books

In the early days, I was much more prone to express my
frustration than Beryl was to express hers. But, in the recorded
interview in 2005, she was quite explicit:

> but more and more I think about these things, and that all these
> things are things that I think about very much now in my mind,
> because now I can't read books. And I can't read, that's the
> hardest thing for me now that I can't do that, and I can't write,
> and things like that and I find it puzzling in many ways but over
> time you get more and more ... cross or horrible and wild about
> those things.

School books

We still have, in our house, several poetry books that Beryl used at school, with her name written in large cursive script, and with 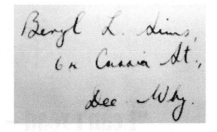 some passages marked with pencil.

She told me, many years ago, about a special poem she knew from school, and I found a copy for her. The poem was called *High Flight,* and was well known in its time.[19] It was written by John Gillespie Magee in 1941, just a few months before he died aged nineteen in an accident in a Spitfire over Lincolnshire. Its youthful simplicity understandably touched the hearts of adolescent schoolgirls, as well as many others around the world. Its fundamental idea is consonant with the ideas, and the more tersely expressed words, of Robert Browning, to which I will refer later in the context of music and meaning.

> *Oh! I have slipped the surly bonds of Earth …*
> *.. with silent, lifting mind I've trod*
> *The high untrespassed sanctity of space*

Beryl's sense of aspiration faced many challenges over the years, but she loved flying until the end.

Poetry and psalms

Before we were married, Beryl showed me one of her books from university about modern poetry, called *Feet on the ground*.[20] I remember it well, and that copy from the 1950s is still on our bookshelves. Another special poem she referred to was by Edith Sitwell: *Still falls the rain*, written after the London blitz in 1940.[21] The poem is dark, and had impressed itself on her during her university years, which began less than ten years after the end of the war.

During the thirty years before her stroke, Beryl introduced me to a wide variety of poets, some less mainstream than others. She referred to Edwin Muir and RS Thomas, and we especially enjoyed tackling Gerard Manley Hopkins together. In Hong Kong, in the 1980s, we experimented with a group in using some of Hopkins' words as a focus during meditation: *dearest freshness deep down things*.[22] After her stroke, Beryl would still look with me at Muir and Thomas and Hopkins. I would read poems, or parts of poems, to her and she would thank me and nod agreement. I mean that she would agree that they were important for her, and not entirely forgotten.

One special discovery of Beryl's was the Russian Irina Ratushinskaya, writing from prison in the 1980s where she was detained for 'anti-Soviet agitation and propaganda' in the form of writing poetry. One poem had struck Beryl particularly, and it related especially to her experiences in the later years after the stroke, with the writer thanking people who were remembering her.[23]

During the ten years before her stroke, Beryl became increasingly absorbed with several small books by Jim Cotter, a poet-priest who was a self-acknowledged depressive. The books were mostly paraphrases of the psalms. After the stroke she continued, almost to the end, to look at these books, many passages of which she marked in pencil with her unsteady left hand. Beryl also watched with me a DVD of Jim Cotter reading many of the poems of RS Thomas on the Llyn peninsula in northwest Wales, where both Thomas and Cotter had lived and worked.[24]

In all the reading described in this chapter, there was, for Beryl, a problem of concentration and continuity, but the fundamental problem was recognising and processing words, including speaking them. I often felt that she enjoyed poetry in all its forms more than prose (fiction or non-fiction), precisely because it was up to her to take the meaning from the words and, in good post-modern style, her own meaning was what mattered rather than anybody else's. And that meaning did not need to be spoken aloud.

Bookshelves and feminist heroines

From her university days, Beryl had a passion for Virginia Woolf's writing. *To the Lighthouse* and *Mrs Dalloway* were her favourites. On the day that her stroke occurred, Beryl was reading Hermione Lee's biography[25] of Virginia Woolf, and the bookmark stayed undisturbed half-way through the book for several years. Beryl would have read Lee's quotation from Woolf's essay *The Humane Art*,[26] commending Horace Walpole: "A self that goes on changing is a self that goes on living." Woolf maintained that only Walpole's unworthy critics said that "his mind was a bundle of inconstant whims and affectations".

Beryl was always as interested in change as I was, and she tolerated my whims. Having warmly embraced and bookshelved George Eliot (Mary Ann Evans) and the Brontë sisters, Beryl moved into reading about women's issues, especially in the context of what can be broadly described as spirituality.

Beryl remembered some of the books which were most significant to her, and which were still all on the bookshelves, even though she could not really say the names of the books, much less read them. Two very special books were entitled *Bread not Stone*[27] (the challenge of feminist biblical interpretation) and *Texts of Terror*[28] (horrific biblical stories with women as victims).

Writing

The last cursive writing of Beryl's that we have is her notes from the day before her stroke. She attended a whole day course on Quaker spirituality; that was the last-but-one session in her two-year training programme as a 'spiritual director' i.e. a listener-confidant-counsellor. Beryl's cursive writing never returned.

ALI

30

I LOVE

YOU

MUM

She did manage, with her non-dominant left hand, on a few occasions to write a few words, and later even a signature in printed capitals and her initials, for example on the forms for power of attorney.

She wrote the birthday card on the left to our daughter seven months after the stroke and, eight months later, she managed to choose and write on a birthday card for

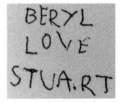

BERYL
LOVE
STUA.RT

me (on the right). I think the word order followed her train of thought (from-to) rather than a traditional to-from format.

But after that she did not write any words at all for more than ten years. She did, however, mark some of her books, highlighting passages that meant something to her, with her unsteady pencil.

Watching

The perceptive speech and language therapist helpfully pointed out quickly that Beryl was a very visual person. Part of her enjoyment of reading was holding the book, looking at the pages and turning them.

Beryl was always a watcher, and she articulated this herself in the interview:

> After the children were grown up, I could do all my ideas what I wanted to do, I could do this or that – everything; but now I'm... we have to wait because there are certain times where I'm just sitting in a corner or... but I... so it's wonderful here now because I watch other things [from the window?]...
>
> Looking back now all these years I can know that I was a person who was always watching other people and paying attention to 'why'

So we frequently watched the television together, often using DVDs. She had read more Tolstoy than I had, and most of EM Forster. For many hours, she watched with me *War and Peace*, *Anna Karenina*, *A Room with a View* and *Howards End*. She watched some repeatedly, especially *Brideshead Revisited*, which we had seen in Hong Kong when it was first shown. Shakespeare plays on DVD were too long for her to concentrate.

But we watched the cinema version of *The Merchant of Venice* a number of times, enhanced by the several visits to Venice we were able to make during the years after the stroke, the last being in November 2014. She loved the BBC programme *Casualty*, but even that became too complicated and lengthy for her. And there was always *Songs of Praise*.

I had taken her occasionally to the cinema, and to a variety of touring opera company performances. She enjoyed those, even though she had sometimes had enough by the interval. She was always happy to go for dinner first. In the last year or two, I took her to some ballet performances locally, and we found excellent ballet programmes on the television that we could watch repeatedly. I never worked out quite why it took me so long to act on my knowledge that ballet had been one of her first loves, and to find suitable occasions for her to watch. I had been distracted by vocal and instrumental music, I guess.

Talking and reading together

I have probably never been a great one for small talk, and before Beryl's stroke, we could be comfortable sitting together or separately with our own thoughts. But that was, more often than not, with a book or a magazine or a notepad in our hands. After the stroke, the dynamic changed because Beryl did not have the books, magazines and notepads to hand.

She remarked in the interview, speaking about me:

> ... some days he's just ... his mind is thinking about other things,
> you know, and I'll feel, 'Oh, well why don't you talk with me?'
> But after a while I got the idea that I'd be sensible and give him
> time ... things like that. But you know over time I think we're a
> bit better than we used to be but I'm not sure... but he doesn't
> say. He'll have to say what he wants to say...

After Beryl's stroke, many people mentioned or sent audio books for her to use and enjoy. However, Beryl had never enjoyed listening to cassettes of talks, and she would not even try most of the (fortunately small) number of audio books that arrived in the house. So, to keep her involved with books, I found as many suitable art books as I could, especially about women artists.

But I also felt that we should try reading together. This approach was not just a substitute for talking or chatting; I hoped it would help and promote our informal talking. I started reading aloud to her from newspapers and magazines, but it was an unfamiliar way of relating both to Beryl and to texts. Beryl made several comments in her interview that relate to this.

> Stuart sometimes will read the Guardian, and he'll talk about
> things and sometimes you are able to do things in detail that I
> love to listen to things....

> Yes, things like that, you see, but on the whole after a while I did
> find it was very hard why he had to do that but he at least listens
> and tells me things that are such a joy really because I can't ...

Having settled into our new house, about five years after the stroke, I finally felt strong enough to tackle reading books to Beryl. This seemed an entirely different enterprise from listening to a recording of someone else reading.

The very first book that I tried reading out loud to Beryl was *The Curious Incident of the Dog in the Night-Time* by Mark Haddon, which had only recently been published.[29] I have to admit that I skipped all the chapters about mathematics. I found them fascinating but Beryl needed to get on with the story. But in the first of the mathematical chapters (chapter 19) I read a view of life which I felt that, in our circumstances at the time, had not been convincingly refuted by any philosophers or theologians whom I have read: that life was like prime numbers, with no patterns that you could work out.

The whole exercise of reading that book was a great success; Beryl seemed wonderfully empathetic to all the characters, especially young Christopher. We moved onto Bill Bryson's *A Sunburned Country* (also know as *Down Under*) and *Notes from a Small Island,* and she had many memories of, or resonances with, parts of both. Then we moved onto more serious matters, including Karen Armstrong's three autobiographical books,[30] one of which Beryl had read in Hong Kong in the 1980s.

So then, I plucked up courage to try reading Virginia Woolf aloud. I started *A Room of One's Own,* as it is straightforward and short, and the only one of her books which I can say I have read in its entirety. But Beryl was not interested; she wanted her favourites. So we started *To the Lighthouse.* However, the first sentence continued from the first page onto the second page, so I simply gave up then and there. After a break, we tried *Mrs Dalloway.* It shared much the same fate. Some years later Beryl watched the film version of *Mrs Dalloway,* with Vanessa Redgrave, right through, with obvious enjoyment and without interruption or comment, on more than one occasion.

Over the years, we read snippets together, focusing more and more on watching things together.

Reading and joining in

From a few years after the stroke, while we were driving to visit our children and their families, it became obvious that Beryl could make out and understand some of the words on road signs, especially the large white-on-blue motorway signs. She would read out loud, with pleasure, the name 'Nottingham', which meant that we were getting close to where the little granddaughters lived.

She could also read words on shopping lists. I printed out a customised version so that she could mark items that she thought we needed.

I have already noted that she could read enough to mark passages in some of her small books, especially poetic works. However, by contrast with the place names on road signs, she could not read out loud the words that she marked. We tried once in the meditation group we were members of. People took turns to bring a short reading, and with my help Beryl chose a few sentences. But she was unable to read them; interestingly, however, she tried to paraphrase what she took to be the import of the words on the paper. We resorted to asking her to choose a painting to bring to the group.

Beryl kept on trying with books; she loved to have them around, and would turn pages keenly. In the first few years after her stroke, she tried very hard to find passages in books which she remembered as relevant to other people – for my mother, when my father died, and for a friend of our own age from many years ago, whose husband had died. She pored over the books, trying to explain to me what she was looking for, and we found what she wanted.

Over the last few years, she relied more and more on books of art or illustration. We found a large print version of *Mrs Dalloway* and it became a good example of her persistent life with books. She loved to sit with it, and with other favourite books, turning a few pages, sometimes clutching them and carrying them. The collections of words meant the world to her, even though she could not read them individually.

Over the years since the stroke, Beryl enjoyed attending our local parish church about once a month, because there seemed to be enough words in one hour in church to last Beryl for a month. But, ten years after the stroke, she started, for the first time after all those years, to try to follow the words of hymns or the liturgy, and join in. I was surprised and delighted. She never managed to join in very much or to keep up, but it was a good experience for both of us. She reminded me sometimes of Lance-Corporal Jones in *Dad's Army*, who was always a little behind everyone else.

A moment of special poignancy was one day when the *Agnus Dei* was read together. This was as recent as September 2014, when her confusion and loss of memory were well established. She tried to follow along, and when everyone had finished I heard her little voice say, quite alone, "Grant us peace." I did not join in anything else for a while, with moist eyes and a lump in my throat.

On our last visit to Australia together, we were able to get to Perth, and with other friends we met two of the people she had begun work with there fifty years previously. One of those friends had just published her mother's life story, and Beryl was delighted to be able to bring a copy home.

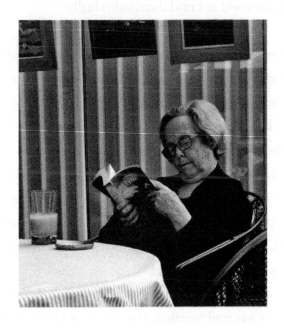

The photograph shows Beryl in our garden room, looking at the book that was titled *One Uncommon Woman*. She looked at the words, usually returning repeatedly to the first few pages. She knew who had written the book, and she knew what it was about, because I had read some of it to her. So she repeatedly enjoyed the experience of holding and being involved with the book. She seemed to absorb some of the meaning and significance of the book without necessarily registering the individual words.

7

"They're all memories that I just keep in my mind"

Bad dreams and bad memories

In the rehabilitation unit, in the weeks after Beryl's stroke, she did not sleep well, and the staff tried several sedatives to help her sleep. However, the first few caused sleep disturbance and nightmares rather than helping. It is interesting that Beryl somehow managed to communicate that she was having bad dreams, despite her severe limitation with words at that stage.

Bad memories have plagued her over the years, more often than not relating to her father's work accident when she was only seven years old. That experience of her father, and thus the experiences of her family and of herself, shaped her life. She spent much of her life before we were married in a part-time caring role. The social context was regrettably often critical and judgemental, and that contributed to the bad memories.

However, on the positive side she became a strong female leader, a sort of proto-feminist.

In the years after the stroke, those bad memories surfaced repeatedly.

To sleep, perchance

Both of us have suffered from chronic sleep disturbance. Beryl's was caused by her brain damage, on top of a tendency to insomnia over the years, while mine was related mainly to being disturbed by her restlessness from drug side effects, or from her illness and insomnia.

In the few years before Beryl's stroke, I became involved with the health services in several prisons in the south of England. One striking fact was the great demand from prisoners for sleeping tablets. Their daily routine was not tiring, and sleeplessness was a major problem. It took only a little questioning to discover the fundamental nature of the problem. It was only when prisoners were asleep that they were not in prison; that is, they were not conscious of being in prison. They wanted oblivion rather than the experience of being in prison.

I have found myself feeling much the same, sometimes to my shame or embarrassment. Increasingly, over the years, it has only been when she has been asleep that I could feel free to write or even watch television, or just to do nothing.

At the same time, when Beryl was able to sleep she could escape from the limitations of her illness, unless the bad dreams and bad memories intruded. As time went by, the amount of sleep, or its value, gradually diminished. I would be glad when she would go to lie down in the daytime but, as the illness progressed, it was rare that this sleep or rest lasted for any length of time. Increasingly, she would get up early in the morning, with the comment, "It's time." It was not actually time for anything in particular, just for the next thing.

Bad judgement

It seems harsh to say that Beryl's judgement became impaired. That may be very subjective for me, and some friends objected on her behalf when I said something along these lines.

When I was small, my mother used to refer sometimes to people "who didn't have enough sense to come in out of the rain." Beryl did not always register that it was raining. I am slightly embarrassed to add that in our community, as we grew up, there were families described as having a child who "wasn't all there". Although I heard the latter phrase used again very recently by a contemporary of mine, both these comments seem politically incorrect in the twenty-first century. But they are both honest observations made without malice. Beryl lost skills; her good judgement, for example, about choosing clothes, not just for matching styles and colours but also for the weather. And Beryl herself remarked later, about some women she met, "Some are not all there."

From the time of the stroke, Beryl lost a coherent grasp of numbers, and thus frequently of costs. I accept full responsibility for spending our money, but we do have a few luxury items that she chose which she would not have done if her memory of costs and values had been retained.

Good memories

Nearly five years after Beryl's stroke, we spent the New Year break with friends in Staffordshire. While driving home Beryl said, entirely out of the blue, "I think we should go and live in Southampton." We had spent the years since the stroke in Rustington, in West Sussex, but in response to Beryl I said, "OK," and we found a new house within two weeks. We both had good memories of Southampton, having lived there with growing children in the 1970s. The facts that she suffered the stroke while visiting our son there, and that he and his family still lived there, were not explicitly mentioned in our decision to move; it was more about old friends of ours, and familiarity with the place.

So some of Beryl's memories and judgements have been good. Quite recently, while driving back from a visit to the

New Forest, we passed a tower block of flats that we must have passed dozens of times. But, on this occasion, she said, entirely spontaneously, something about "those ladies living there". I had to rack my brains about that remark, and eventually realised that some of the women who clean for us did live there when we first discussed the matter more than five years previously. I have no recollection of the topic ever being discussed again. So, memories are still there, and I wondered about the comparison: is my memory the standard by which I measure hers?

Remembered activities and people

Especially in looking through photograph albums, and the life story books that we have assembled for her, Beryl has remembered people and places. It has seemed ironic that as life and the effects of her illnesses progressed, and as Beryl depended more and more on her memory, the memory was fading. She tended to remember people and places from a long time ago, such as friends from Western Australia in the 1960s and the school she taught at in Hong Kong in the 1980s. She remembered activities in London from just before the stroke less well – although they could be prompted by photographs – such as being a steward at the Globe Theatre, and being involved with Jubilee 2000, and with the development agency Shared Interest in Newcastle-upon-Tyne.

One of Beryl's friends from her school days kept in touch with us over the years. Up until the last time we met, a couple of years ago, the friend could raise a smile from Beryl by recounting tales of school, for example of a very perky Beryl announcing, "I have arrived" when she burst in late to a lesson in secondary school. These were memories that I did not share, along with memories of her early family ups and downs.

Remembered abilities, and forgotten ones

In the recorded interview, Beryl was very aware of the changes in our roles and activities in the household.

> I'm aware that I can't do everything, and that's because maybe Stuart's the person who has done much more of the hard work, you know, when he is helping me. And I'm just so used now that he does all the cooking, which is amazing, and things like that ...

She would sometimes become distressed by her memories of what she had been able to do. Since we moved back to London in the late 1990s, Beryl was never particularly interested in driving. She enjoyed making full use of the public transport in London, and taking the train whenever it was feasible.

But, not much more than a year ago, she was still sometimes distressed by not doing 'her' jobs; she notably looked on while I did the ironing, not that I did more than the basics. Her distress was not about the change of roles – that never bothered her. She was always pleased for me to do the cooking, and the shopping too. What distressed her was the awareness that she was no longer capable of coping with a hot iron, or a hot oven, or a supermarket.

In relation especially to activities of daily living, Beryl and some other stroke sufferers have had a form of forgetfulness that is not related to memory in the sense that we normally use the word. 'Sensory inattention' is the term used to describe a change in the ability to feel things, for example when holding them. It is not that the hand has lost its capacity to feel; there is no 'anaesthesia', as it were. The problem is that the feelings do not seem to register in the usual way; 'inattention' seems to be just the right word.

Beryl never lost her willingness, her desire, to be helpful. She had been accustomed to making and having a tidy house. Although I think I did well at maintaining that ideal, it did happen that frequently she wanted to tidy up, partly because my time frame was not always the same as hers. But there was a problem when she picked up, for example, a cup in her right hand. Her right arm was weak ever since the stroke, and had lost the fine movements needed for writing and so on, as opposed to the so-called coarse movements. She could pick up an empty cup with her right hand, a full one being heavy as well as dangerous. But she could not do anything useful with the cup; even place it down reliably. The problem from the sensory inattention was that her brain seemed to 'forget' that the cup was there in her hand. It is understandable that I would fuss, especially about her carrying things in either hand while going up and down the stairs at home, even though we are used to having several flights of stairs in our houses. I have to acknowledge, however, that she only dropped and broke two cups in all the years after the stroke. As I emphasised to her, the breaking of the cup was of no consequence in itself. The problem was that she might fall or hurt herself in the process.

Tidying up clothes was less dangerous, but if she carried them with her right arm or hand, they were likely to fall and be left behind with her quite unaware. This carried over into getting dressed. Since the stroke, she became less and less able to dress herself. The sensory inattention and weakness of the right arm were a major part of this problem, although she became increasingly unsure and muddled about the whole business as time went by.

About three years after the stroke, we managed to make our first visit to the Holy Island of Lindisfarne in the north east of England. A taxi took us back to the train as we were leaving. In the taxi, I took stock of us and of our belongings. Beryl had been helping by holding a carrier bag, but it became apparent that the bag of items for the journey, including our camera, had been left by the roadside as we had waited and then got into the taxi. Sensory inattention is not necessarily a disastrous problem, but it needs to be managed, and that can be difficult without the carer appearing to be directive or censorious, and the sufferer (for want of a better word) being made to feel like a child.

Socialising has always been important for us, including eating out, especially with friends. With Beryl's sensory inattention, and with her having to eat using her non-dominant hand, which has mild arthritis, we have often looked for finger food. Most restaurants seem accustomed to dealing with, and helping, eccentric or disabled older people, and even the upmarket places do not seem offended if such adults eat with their fingers. But Beryl did sometimes verbalise her objection to being treated like a child, for example if I asked her to slow down as she was eating. It was not part of what the family call her 'pre-morbid personality' to fill up her mouth like a hamster, but her awareness was not what it used to be.

Interests and options

I can remember asking Beryl from time to time, and in various contexts including both big issues and small ones, what she wanted to do. I accepted her frequent answer that she did not know, although I did not always understand. But in the years after her stroke, with the restrictions that affected both of us, I came to experience what she meant. For example, a friend asked me, "Stuart, what are you going to do when Beryl dies?" I can remember laughing involuntarily, and saying, "How do you expect me to answer that sort of question?" I was learning that there are some questions about interests and options that cannot be answered, because in some situations there are, or seem to be, simply no conceivable options.

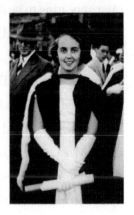

There was, however, one thing that Beryl had really wanted to do: what used to be called 'personnel management'. She had applied for a training post from University but was told to come back when she looked older.

Beryl at graduation aged nineteen

In the recorded interview, Beryl described her interests as remembered strongly from nearly fifty years before, but she could not remember the words 'personnel management':

> I was so puzzled at that time that looking back now all these years I can know that I was a person who was always watching other people and paying attention to 'why', what's wrong with people in my mind, it was a sort of ... and I know I wanted to be a... the first time when I was very young I wanted to be into...now the words ... I wanted to be a ... I didn't really want to become a

teacher, but I knew I wanted to be a person who can talk about other people, like, ... *[Stuart prompts: Personnel Management]* Yes. That's the sort of thing because I liked to have people who wanted to talk about this work, and then I helped them, how you can do this and that and the other, and you know, that sort of thing but I was very, very young. Early on. And I knew that was my calling, that I would have been if I'd had time ...

She also remembered, clearly, the disappointment at having (after twenty years, not forty as she said in the interview below) managed to obtain a qualification in personnel management but then not been able to use it. This was because we went, with her full agreement, to Hong Kong, and she discovered that the language barrier was insurmountable.

Forty years later on I had a go and got into that work. But, except, the day I got all those bits and bobs to say, you know, I would be allowed to do it, everything, then I had to go to Hong Kong; and it gave me six months before my brain thought that that was, I can't realise, oh of course I can't say it, Chinese?

They're all memories

It has been ironic that, as input from written material decreased, it followed that life depended more on memory, while at the same time the memory continued to fade. That involved all the types of memory that the experts describe; short term and long term and other classifications.

A classic example was in the car. She has asked repeatedly where we are going. When repeating the answer, it has seemed to me that this was not just a short-term memory problem. It was as though my answer was never properly heard. Perhaps that it was never even listened to; as though the answer never got into any sort of memory at all. Perhaps it was as if she was not really asking a question so much as expressing unease or confusion. I could not always distinguish the effects of the initial stroke from the effects of increasing age and progressive brain disease.

In the interview she said:

> Anyhow, all those things, they're all memories that I just keep in my mind.

But, more and more, the memories were not kept in her mind.

Those blue remembered mountains

We both grew up in the 1940s and 1950s in Sydney, where the area called the Blue Mountains was fifty miles inland to the west. We learnt in school about Blaxland, Lawson and Wentworth, who first found a way over those mountains in 1813, opening up the enormous plains further west, while in Europe groups such as the Luddites, and Napoleon's armies, were causing and having their own problems. I had my seventh birthday at a holiday cottage in the Blue Mountains. There was a brushing of snow; the first I had ever seen. As a child, Beryl went on a steam train to visit relatives who lived in the foothills, and she also told me of the happy times she had with university friends, and their families, in holiday houses up on the mountains.

But that is all a long time ago. In his poem *A Shropshire Lad*,[31] (located about half-way between our time and Napoleon's) AE Housman wrote of the feelings that Beryl so often reflected: of *those blue remembered hills* which, in the poem, represented

> *... the land of lost content ...*
> *The happy highways where I went*
> *And cannot come again.*

Beryl barely remembered the Blue Mountains. Certainly, much of her contentment was lost. There were many places where neither her body nor her mind could come again.

8

Lost for words – reflections written in 2004

Carers and creative writing

Soon after Beryl suffered the stroke, we retreated from central London to the village of Rustington. Through the community stroke rehabilitation team, and through contacts in the NHS where I managed to work part-time, I became involved in a variety of groups and activities for carers in the area. They were support groups, and a form of rehabilitation for me in my new circumstances and roles. One of the carers had set up a creative writing group, and I joined that a few years after the stroke.

Words fail me – and her, and us

I wrote the following lines in March 2004, more than ten years ago. They were written out of frustration, and reflection, and a desire for greater fluency than was possible at home. Despite the time, and the deterioration over the years, many of the sentiments have stayed as relevant as ever.

Words Fail Me

Words fail me.
I am speaking, of course, for her
But that is not what she really wants
And I often used to interrupt her – even speak for her
Before the stroke
Even though I was signed up to feminist principles as much as she was.

But if I were to speak for her
(And sometimes – frequently – now she asks me to)
I would say that names and numbers are the words that
   really faze me
But that's me breaking in again with one of my wisecracks.
"Aphasia" is what I have (she says)
(Hence my 'faze' joke)
(Who's doing the talking here – I keep taking over when she's
   speaking?)
Aphasia - where words won't and don't come to mind or
   come out right

Especially when I'm weary or stressed or taken by surprise.

I used to read and write and talk and advise and counsel –
even preach!

And although I had learnt to be quiet and still and to listen,

Nevertheless the words were part of what I was.

And now words fail me

And it's the inability to get words in by reading and out by writing

which is more devastating than the inability to speak the words.

Words fail me – but sometimes I can't help feeling

(Because I was brought up in a context of judgement and
blame – especially of myself)

That in fact I fail the words.

Words fail us.

We were advised – warned – about how difficult negotiation would be

And that's just one of the innumerable helpful inputs from the
wonderful therapist

Who came to support her – and us.

Could two frustrated people possibly be better than one frustrated
person?

Perhaps in as much as they (we) keep talking – or trying to talk

Maybe after a break – even a walk

Or a glass of something – but careful with the drugs she's taking,

Moderate alcohol only!

Sometimes words do go right –

And can be praised (can that be right?)

"Accolade" — that was one of her really good words early on,

The very first however being "organise"

And we can laugh about that

And when we don't feel unwell we can manage laughs

And good chats with children and grandchildren

And even newer acquaintances.

It's not all bad, we sometimes think.

Words fail us — but not all the time

And occasionally the slightly wrong word makes us all laugh together!

So do words fail me? (This is me.)

I'm doing quite well with these words now that I've got started.

Getting started with writing has never been very easy, even with writing for work.

Often I'm not sure what I really think — there are too many possibilities.

However, in the context of chronic illness and disability and dysphasia

But also in the context of a meditation group that we have both joined recently

And of the Quaker meeting which I have joined,

Perhaps there is much for me in the quiet

And it's not always and entirely a negative thing when

Words fail me.

Lost for words – me, her, us, everyone?

I wrote the next piece in December 2004, but it seems like yesterday. The experiences I recorded have remained accurate descriptions of everyday life, even more so as time and deterioration have progressed. The temptation, or inclination, to give up on words and just do the thing – to, about, or with her, or even without her – persisted; even increased. And when I wrote the piece, the added dimensions of the problem, the confusion and loss of memory, were still to come. But they were coming.

Lost for words

I am lost for words.
You (singular) are lost for words.
He, she or it is lost for words.
We are lost for words.
You (plural) are lost for words.
They are lost for words.

In Latin I learnt to conjugate verbs (as I have just done for "lost") and to decline nouns. But now all words are declining, have declined, will decline – now I'm on to tense. And tense is what it often is.

I often think it is like trying to converse in a language in which one is not fluent – the draining effort of trying to translate as one goes along, the ease of some parts not compensating for the frustration of the difficult parts – often the most important parts.

For the most part, 'she is lost for words' is the situation. During one of her admissions to hospital I 'helpfully' explained to the medical student clerking her that she was a textbook case of 'nominal aphasia' that we all learn about in medical school. It really is quite astonishing how what gets lost are the names of things – real concrete things more noticeably than abstractions. Grammar gets a bit shaky; irregular verbs can be a problem, which is one of the many aspects that prompt thoughts about growing grandchildren and how they will develop and move on to greater competence, while Gran won't.

Of course sometimes 'they' are lost for words. It is really helpful (I don't think) when presumably well-meaning but actually ignorant acquaintances remark how they too often forget names or words – it's part of growing older. No, it damn well isn't – not this sort of loss of words.

And me – the wordsmith – do I get lost for words? Not much, but I am getting better at it! I mean that I am learning to let the words go, to listen to the silence, to let the wordy thoughts run down, to meditate or muse. But the words keep flowing, and (in

common, I am told, with many carers of people with aphasia)
after 6 or 12 months I gradually stopped feeling guilty about
having retained some facility with words, reading especially.
Textbooks don't have a fancy expression in Greek or Latin (or
what one of my anatomy teachers used to call a bastardised
combination of both) for loss of ability to take in words from
written texts. Illiteracy isn't considered a medical problem
— but loss of 'literacy' (which dictionaries define to include
both reading and writing) is a profound problem, especially
for those whose life and work was based on written words.
So we are lost for words, you the reader and I, she and I. I am told
that many languages including ancient Greek have a proverb
to the effect that 'actions speak louder than words'. So that
is the way we go, separately and together, doing as well as
speaking. We have been challenged over the years about the
importance of 'being' as well as or rather than 'doing'. We are
learning to go that way too.

These words from 2004 became the basis of this book, and of
its companion that follows. In the companion book, there are a
few more short pieces, one about 'spirituality with few words'.
That particular piece became memorable to me because it was
published, and through a coincidence of circumstances brought
Beryl, and thus me, into contact with a friend and colleague
whom she had not met for forty years, and who was very

supportive of both of us. I have also included a short published piece from 2011 in the companion book. It relates to labyrinths, to which I refer in a later chapter about images.

"I thought she might have dementia"

Not the D word, please

At about the time the two pieces in the previous chapter were written, I attended a public meeting in our village related to the part-time NHS work with which I was involved. I took Beryl, and an experienced colleague met her for the first time.

The next day I met the colleague, who said that she was not sure about the nature of Beryl's health problems. She said, "I thought she might have dementia." I can remember feeling immediately offended at the suggestion, on Beryl's behalf. But it might have also been on my own behalf, and I can remember thinking at the same time what an extraordinary reaction it was on my part. It confirmed, in my experience, what I had known well in theory for twenty-five years: the powerful reality of *labelling* and the associated *stigma*. Just the word 'dementia' was enough, then, to raise all sorts of issues in my mind.

I make no claim to virtuous political correctness here. I remember talking with friends and family about how Beryl managed in the local shops. I casually said something like, "In this village, the shops are used to dealing with daft old bats." I cringe now at the idea that I must have felt that using words like "daft" and calling older women "old bats" were somehow much more commonplace and acceptable than a more-or-less-technical word like dementia. And, of course, it was true that there were similarities then between Beryl's appearance and behaviour and that of people suffering from dementia.

Learning about mental health and mental illness

When I was a medical student there was, in the community, still considerable ambivalence and uncertainty about mental illness, and about psychiatry and its practitioners. In the general hospital where I trained, the reputation of the specialty was not helped by the observation one day of a consultant psychiatrist walking across the road outside the hospital carrying an axe. His reputation for being odd, or even 'mad', seemed justified.

But at the same time we had some brilliant teachers in psychiatry. With as much sensitivity as skill, they could interview patients with florid psychoses in front of a group of a hundred students, for example a young woman who thought she was the Virgin Mary. In a similar context, one rather suave professor remarked, not unkindly, that the situation seemed "beyond the bounds of religious eccentricity".

Not so many years later, Beryl suffered from profound perinatal depression, made worse by complicated hormonal therapy and prolonged prenatal hospitalisation. We learnt together how to live with mental health problems, and also what it meant to be 'users' of mental health services.

So, all in all, I had no good reason to be sensitive about Beryl having a label of dementia. But I guess it felt like an added complication, and an added burden both for her already challenging life and for my life, on top of the stroke. And that was the reality.

Getting lost

I described earlier the extraordinary way in which, soon after the stroke, Beryl got herself from our apartment in London to our house in Rustington. I realise that although, in a sense, on that occasion I lost her, she herself was not lost. However, things began to change. In our new locality in Southampton she could, for some years, find her way over some distance, even to the local shops. But then one day I really did lose her; it was the first of many occasions.

She was never particularly a wanderer, but Charles de Gaulle airport in Paris was probably a special case. Checking in with my sister, we realised that Beryl simply was not there. This was 2008, and Beryl's confusion was beginning to show itself in a different way from previously. The airport check in area was enormous but, fortunately, she had gone on walking in a straight line after we turned aside. I found her in a few minutes, but it was an anxious time.

Within those few years, changes occurred which made me realise that her situation was beginning to move in what I cannot help thinking of as that dreaded direction. Memories had been disturbed, as I have described, and she could also seem confused because of her problems with words. But, eventually, it was apparent that further specialist assessment was needed in order to try to help with her problems in daily living.

Keep C-A-L-M and carry on?

I tried to find other ways of talking and writing about these problems, partly because, in principle, I did not like the D word for dementia. I felt that it was not a particularly descriptive or meaningful word in discussing her problems, either with Beryl herself or with other people, whether involved in health care or not.

One day I thought of what I might call a reverse acronym: CALM standing for Confusion, Agitation and Loss of Memory.

That is as good a short description as one can get, I think, of the whole picture of dementia. But, as an acronym, it is either too clever by half, or just too perverse, to be useful.

And so our excellent local NHS general practitioner, who had got to know Beryl well, agreed with me that specialist assessment was needed, with a view to getting the best advice about the management of Beryl's problems.

Assessment

It was at the end of 2010 when Beryl was referred to what was called the Memory Clinic, which I thought was a good label. After a home visit, we went to the hospital for an outpatient appointment. I was rather put out when the nurse insisted that I leave Beryl with her for the complicated verbal and visual assessment. This was partly based on earlier experiences with some health professionals, but in the event all went well. Beryl was content and the nurse was clearly extremely competent.

Beryl had a number of blood tests, and then an MRI scan. We (I say 'we' automatically because that was how it felt) ended up with a diagnosis of mainly 'vascular dementia', with possibly minor Alzheimer's changes also. The precise diagnosis was not entirely a theoretical matter, because the drugs available with possible benefits were tested on, and licensed for, Alzheimer's disease; a specific illness that causes dementia.[32]

Vascular dementia[33] is the second most common type of dementia in the United Kingdom after Alzheimer's disease, affecting around 150,000 people, about one-fifth of the total. Vascular dementia is caused by reduced blood supply to the brain. This can be due to diseased blood vessels, or to single or repeated small blood clots, and is not uncommon after a stroke. Vascular dementia is uncommon under age 65, and specific risks are previous stroke, diabetes or heart disease.

It was therefore not unexpected that Beryl was diagnosed with vascular dementia. But, because of the possibly mixed picture, the Memory Clinic agreed to give Beryl a trial period with one of the anti-Alzheimer's drugs. The major effect was, however, six weeks of sleep disturbance with no noticeable changes of memory or confusion, so the drug was stopped.

Beryl was kept under review, and later it was possible to try other drugs. Mostly, however, the challenge was to cope with sleep disturbance from the illness rather than from drugs, and with agitation. We benefited from on-going care and support from the primary care team, and also from the so-called Admiral Nurses, who have a very specialised capability and who work with families and carers in the context of dementia.[34]

A consumer's view of research

As a former editor of an international epidemiology journal, I am well aware of the temptations and the pitfalls of studies of associations between diseases and possible risk factors in large groups of people in the community. When it comes to postulating causal mechanisms, the imagination of researchers seems unlimited.

That is well illustrated by a comment of Beryl's sister, whose husband was being cared for with dementia in Canberra, Australia. Yet another research report had been published about the causes of Alzheimer's disease. This time the report was that people with Blood Group O (which applies to nearly half of many populations) had a *lower* risk. Beryl's sister said, "It is just a joke," and I am inclined to agree.

It is true, however, that biological research into the causes, and thus possible prevention or limitation of Alzheimer's disease, has advanced. We all hope for further advances and for some real success stories. For people with vascular conditions like Beryl, it is highly unlikely that advances with Alzheimer's will have any benefit at all, but very recent reports suggest that better control of high blood pressure may have a major influence on the occurrence of vascular dementia.[35]

Mind, memories and meaning

"We all forget things." People still sometimes say that to me, and my sense of irritation expressed in my prose poem *Lost for Words* in an earlier chapter does not decrease over time.

In his poem *A Shropshire Lad*,[36] Housman described imagining "the smoke of thought blow clean away" and that seemed sometimes to describe the situation we were in. It is much more than sometimes forgetting things. Sally Magnusson's moving and informative book, a memoir of her mother's experience of dementia, is titled *Where Memories Go*.[37] Many novelists as well as philosophers down the ages have used phrases something like, "We are our memories". Keith Ward, for example, writes that for people to maintain their individuality, the continuous chains of memories and thoughts and feelings seem much more important than bodily continuity.[38]

So can there be meaning in life without memories? I really did not want to think about all this when the question about dementia first arose less than five years after Beryl's stroke. I had no way of knowing then whether or when such problems might arise. But, as time and the illness progressed, this problem became a major focus.

10

"Do you understand what I'm saying?"

What about this?

A simple example of Beryl's dysphasia, and the problems for me or any other listener, is when she said, "What about this thing there?" when *this thing* could be anything at all, unless she was able to point it out. Recently she said, "What about the other one down there?" Initially, she frequently made general remarks about *this, that and the other* or about *bits and bobs*. When she said *up* or *down*, and *left* or *right*, it was unclear what she meant. Sometimes, seemingly the opposite came out, but not dependably or predictably. And it was the same with comprehension; sometimes she understood what I meant when I said *up the stairs* or *down the stairs*, but sometimes she did not. She did not reliably understand which room I mean when I said b*edroom*, or *bathroom* or *kitchen*. Over recent years, her mental confusion made the problem worse.

From the time immediately after the stroke, numbers continued to be quite unreliable, even meaningless. But she did not often need to use numbers. Colours were different. They came into the conversation frequently in a variety of contexts, from cardigans to flowers. The colours she named were hardly ever the same as what other observers would use. Sometimes it seemed as though she might be verbalising the complementary colour; the opposite, as it were. But that was both unreliable and of no practical help. Not so long ago she referred to *those little yellow things we have for lunch*. I frowned for a moment, and then smiled when I worked out that she was talking about small tomatoes, which were the usual tomato-red colour. One time when she was correct, in a way, was during a summer visit to some extensive local gardens; she remarked, "All the colours of the rainbow!"

So we often had to try to guess her meaning from a word or two, vague or incorrect words at that. The initial warning of the speech and language therapist, that negotiation would be difficult, proved to be true and persistent, and this applied to all exchanges, not just complicated negotiations. The whole experience often reminded me of the rather languid mother of a young heroine in one of Sandi Toksvig's novels.[39] The mother's sentences habitually tailed off halfway through, ending with "… et cetera … " where the listeners had to make their own judgement about what was missing. At the same time, there was often something of the scattergun about Beryl's sentences, changing topic halfway through.

Dementia and dysphasia affect words differently

There was a subtle and slow change over the last five years or more, from dysphasia to confusion and then incoherence, all made even more confusing for the listener because the dysphasia was still both present and variable. It has seemed impractical in this book to try to make a precise separation between the problems of dysphasia and dementia developing over time in the one person.

She once said, "It's so dark I can't hear," and on another occasion she said, "I can't see what they're saying". In context, it was not too difficult to understand and act on the remarks – they related to the television. The first time, she meant the sunlight was so bright that she could not see the screen, so we shut the curtains. The second time, the volume was too low. It seems to me that both these instances were essentially a problem of dysphasia rather than dementia.

Other times she had said, "My ring is missing," and "My ring has disappeared again." This was complicated, because her engagement and wedding rings had started to slip off. A year or two previously, we had her wedding ring enlarged because the finger was becoming swollen with arthritis. But, subsequently, all her fingers became thinner again, with general weight loss. So all her rings had recently stayed in their containers to guard against them being lost. What she had been referring to as being missing was, in fact, her watch. We occasionally forgot to put the watch on in the morning. With loss of fine movement in the right hand, she had not been able to put it on and take it off reliably after the stroke. The irony is that for the first few years she was really able to 'tell the time'. She was never able, since the stroke, to say what the time was, but up until the last few years, what she had seen on the watch face obviously had meaning for her in terms of where the day was going. Eventually, she just liked the reassurance of having the watch on her wrist, and could be reluctant to remove it for bed or even for a shower.

A few good words

We visited Sydney about eighteen months after the stroke, and Beryl's speech still had major problems. Family members praised her for her bravery and determination, her efforts and perseverance. Retiring to bed early after one of these family exchanges, she smiled at me as she laid her head on the pillow, and said just the one word: *Accolade*.

Good words, unusual and complicated words, have tended to pop out in unpredictable places. When a new carer came to help, after a session or two Beryl said the carer was *affable*. Beryl was not a great animal lover, but to two little dogs connected with a granddaughter and a niece she recently awarded the epithet of *placid*.

Some of her interesting, less common words have described less than ideal situations. One of the day centres that she attended for a year or so was, Beryl said, *dispiriting*, and the people there were a *motley crew*. One of the care homes at which she stayed for about two weeks was, she said, *torpid*.

Some of her interesting words and ideas did not come out quite right, but expressed clear understanding and insight. Over the years before, and also since, her stroke, Beryl had been a listener to an older woman who had led a remarkable and challenging life.

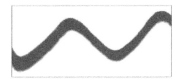

The shape that Beryl traced in the air with her hand

A few years ago, Beryl walked up the stairs towards me at the end of a 45-minute telephone conversation with that woman, a time of listening rather than conversing. As Beryl approached me, she waved her hand in the air, describing the pattern shown in the picture. She said to me, "What's that polar bear thing?" Because I know well the person she had been talking to, it took me just a moment to decipher and translate. She was telling me of her awareness of having just spent a long time listening to the highs and lows of a person with *bipolar disorder*.

But she was perfectly clear and appropriate when she said, after I had been the one having a similarly long phone call, "Too much talking."

At the very least, these 'good words' have indicated to me that Beryl's memory still had much content of an elaborate nature, even if there were major blockages between where the memories were and the outside world. This problem persisted, but the confusion and memory loss complicated her words in other ways as well. For example, it would be less than honest not to note that a few 'bad words' popped out in exceptional circumstances. I never heard her say a four-letter word but, apparently, a care-worker did. This seems to be a common occurrence in dementia, even amongst people with the most buttoned-up of backgrounds, religious or otherwise.

Humour in dysphasia and dementia?

A few years ago, we attended a play at the local university about dementia. To my amazement, Beryl contributed to the discussion afterwards with a comment, although I do not think she was understood by anyone except me. Beryl clearly did not connect herself with the problem under discussion. I asked a question about whether the author had written for laughs, because the audience had laughed at the very stressed reaction of a member of a family trying to cope with parents developing dementia. A response came from a very earnest professional in the audience (who had misunderstood my question), "There is a lot of humour in dementia." I might have been moved to kick her if I had been closer, and I refrained from pointing out that although occasionally we laugh, there is, for the sufferer and the carer, no humour in dementia as an illness.

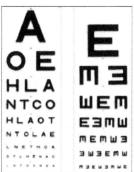

A few years after her stroke, we were pleased that Beryl was continuing to look at books, pictures and words. We agreed that she might benefit from some new reading glasses, so we visited a local optician. We were ushered in to meet a young man who seemed very uncommunicative. I explained that because of the stroke, Beryl would not be able to name the letters reliably on any eye chart, even if she could see them clearly. But the optician appeared to take no notice and asked her to look at the usual chart (the left of the picture). She was confused, and could say nothing. He switched to the E chart (the right of the picture), where she was to say which way the arms of the E were pointing. Beryl's confusion increased. I was feeling more and more irritated, but the optician persisted with little conversation, and showed

Beryl the chart used for children (the next picture), which had the silhouettes of various animals in various sizes. This was beyond her capabilities in so many ways that I had to bite my tongue. The optician silently admitted defeat and dimmed the lights in order to make his assessment by examining Beryl's

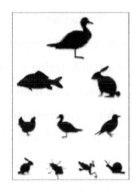

eyes directly with various lighted gadgets. I sat beside Beryl in the dark, with the optician standing in front of her. After a brief pause, Beryl suddenly said, in a loud voice, "Duck." It was a surreal experience. Unless my memory deceives me, I instinctively ducked down in my chair. Of course, Beryl was naming the first animal she saw in the children's chart, after a minute or two of mental processing, the simple version of the pathway being: eye – visual cortex of the brain – various parts of the memory (muddled) – speech centre of the brain (malfunctioning) – voice. I cannot remember any of us laughing at the time, but I have laughed with family and friends when retelling the story.

Occasionally there are little glimpses of humour that may or may not be appreciated by Beryl, as well as those with her. Our first grandchild was eighteen months old when Beryl had the stroke, and they are fond of each other. At age three or four, she was being amusing for Gran and the family, and

Beryl said, "You little mince." We all laughed, but I am not sure that Beryl saw the amusement in the word substitution for *minx* which, ironically, would have been another good word, if slightly old-fashioned. Another time, we had a courtesy car while our own car was being serviced. Beryl remarked that the courtesy car was *itchy*. I realised that she meant *titchy* – that is, tiny.

Sometimes, the humour really is there for her as well as us. Quite recently, we had a very good lunch together at a garden centre, and at home I asked her if she had enjoyed it. Yes, she said, "It was Zero", and then she laughed, remarking, "I've said the wrong thing." Presumably she meant it was 100%, or something like that; we let it go rather than pursue the lost word.

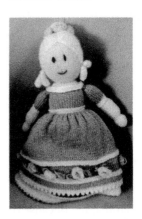

Someone was making soft toys recently and gave one to Beryl. She kept it on her bed, and frequently referred to the little *dog*. The photograph shows how funny her wrong word was. But as I write this I feel that I am perhaps mocking her, mocking the illness, and I feel ashamed. She was not trying to be amusing. However, the problem was her dysphasia rather than her dementia. Nevertheless, is there really 'a lot of humour in dementia'? Mostly, I think not.

Wine nonstop

We had found some new perfumes over the last few years. I gave her a generous spray not long ago, to which she responded, *Lovely fragrance*. So it was not all doom and gloom even if it often, or mostly, seemed to be.

On a summer evening we had ice cream together in our sunny garden room, looking out at the mediaeval city wall and the Tudor Merchant's House, and our colourful little courtyard garden. I brought out a half-bottle of Prosecco, and when I opened it there was a loud "pop". She ducked her head, but as she did so she clearly said *Lovely*.

Then, on one autumn Sunday, we sat again in the sun in our garden room. We had coffee, crispy pancetta on soft bread rolls with small red peppers stuffed with ricotta, followed by bite-sized stollen with a glass of Prosecco. She said she needed to rest, but then noticed that there was more in the bottle and asked for a top-up. I said "Rest first and we'll finish the Prosecco later." She said, "That's very boring."

Another time she was having lunch out with our daughter-in-law, and announced, "I could have wine non-stop." A family joke runs: there's only one thing that Beryl prefers to a glass of champagne – and that is two glasses of champagne. Because of the interaction between alcohol and several of the drugs that she was taking, especially the blood-thinning drug warfarin, it was important that her alcohol intake did not vary widely. We did not have to persuade her to keep it up at a generous level.

Frustration, confusion, insight and sadness

The expressions that Beryl used repeatedly seemed to come from various perspectives. But I cannot fit them into neat categories. Frustration was initially the major issue but, as time passed, confusion was added. Many sayings still seemed based on insight into her predicament. And, frequently, the expressions were also clearly ones of sadness, depression, even despair.

Her frustration came out with expressions like, "I can't do this," and "I can't do that," and "I'm fed up." Nevertheless, she still occasionally said, "I am capable to do that." But mostly her comments related to awareness of loss. She would say, "I can't carry on."

Over the last year or two she repeated, "I feel overwhelmed." She said, "My life is about problems" and "I can't do anything by myself." She would say, "I don't feel whole" and "I am perplexed" and "My mind doesn't work." What I think of as the coup de grâce is, "I'm such a muddled person." Even in this situation, her good humour was not always completely lost. Describing a relative in a care home, she said, "And now he's lost the plot, like me!" and as she said it she laughed with understanding, not confusion.

Such insight and awareness, as she had more often than not, made the particular situation, and life in general, more difficult for both of us rather than easier. One of the unanticipated effects of anti-Alzheimer's drugs, when they were first introduced about twenty years ago, was sometimes to increase awareness, and with the awareness came increased sadness; that also may have been true of Beryl. Once, after the bed linen needed changing several times, she said, "I don't do it out of malice." I do not usually get cross with her in that sort of situation, but that time it was hard not to weep instead. When I was trying to sort out dressing and eating, and outings and jobs around the house, she sometimes said, "Don't shout at me." So I have not always remained cool, calm and clinically detached when faced with the dysphasia, compounded by the dementia. At breakfast she would say, "Can I go upstairs?" When I responded on one occasion, "Can I finish my breakfast?" my voice obviously became louder. "Calm down," she said, "Calm down."

Very frequently, in all sorts of places, including our living room or bedroom or bathroom, she would say, "I want to go home." This saying started right back in the rehabilitation unit, in the first weeks after the stroke, but I was never sure quite what she was meaning. My latest and best guess is that she was referring to the past, possibly to her childhood or young adulthood, when things were as they should be, and she was herself in a way that she was comfortable with, as opposed to now. Indeed, very recently, she said, "I just want to go back to the old days". Perhaps that was her main meaning all the time. At other times, she said, "I just want to be myself; I would like to be what I really am." And she also said, "I just want to go home and do things properly."

One time she added, "I just want to go home – first class!" But mostly it was desperately, heart-rendingly sad to hear her repeat, again and again and again, "I just want to go home."

She became sad quite often, and aware of being unhappy. "All my life was wonderful but now it's all gone off," she said. "I want to be happy; I'm just asking what I could do to be happy." And she compounded my uneasiness by adding, "I'm lonely; I'm on my own," said while I was sitting in the chair next to her. The sadness frequently had a frankly depressive edge to it. I have never been comfortable with the view of some of my conservative psychiatrist acquaintances that suicidal thoughts are necessarily a sign of mental illness. In some cases, including Beryl's, they seem quite rational; that seems like the appropriate word, although I can see that it is perhaps questionable. She said, "I'm fed up with the whole drama," and "Well, what's the point of life?" Also, "I don't like my life" and "Ten o'clock – I'll be dead by that time." Or "Every time I get that horrible feeling that I'll be dead." And she concluded, as it were, "I just feel I've had enough; I just want to go away." It was often hard to disagree. But I have felt lonely too. One of the characters in Shaffer and Barrows' charming novel set in Guernsey reflected on there being nothing lonelier than living the rest of her life with someone she couldn't talk to.[40]

It is burnt into my memory that, forty-five years ago, she was inconsolably sad, with perinatal depression. I mean, literally inconsolable; she would ask me to come to bed and hold her while she sobbed, and I could do nothing else with effect. Medication was, in time, followed by slow improvement. Recently, she had often become not just inconsolably sad, but also incoherently sad. And yet, perhaps, understandably so; this may have been depression, but even more it was an awareness of loss.

Often, Beryl would say, "I don't know where I am," usually when at home. Increasingly she would ask, "Who are they?" when I have mentioned friends or neighbours, and this began to apply to the names of family members, even sometimes to people in photographs. A day or two after she came home from being in hospital with pneumonia, over Christmas 2014, we were sitting together in the lounge. She turned to me and said, "What's your name?" When I said that she knew what my name was, she smiled and said it. That was the only occasion when she said that, but it seemed ominous.

Her restlessness continued to increase, both during the day and at night. She often said, "We had better get going", even in the middle of talking with friends. She wanted to go out, to move on, to do something, or something different. I even had to put a latch on the front door at home because she would let herself out rather than wait for me. "Am I allowed?" she would ask, about shoes and clothes and food and wine. She used to say in the early morning as well as other times, "It's time."

But still trying to converse

Beryl always loved being with the grandchildren and talking with them. She would, in the early days after the stroke, try to read books with them, which meant her making up stories based on the pictures. That did not matter, until the children were old enough to read the words for themselves.

Chatting was less complicated, at least when they were young. Our daughter remarked that when the littlest one was about three years old, she would sit and chat with Gran, and they would each understand about 50% of what the other was saying!

Back in the early days after the stroke, the speech and language therapist talked about Beryl possibly losing some of her inhibitions. I remember replying that I thought that was not likely to affect her speech; that had never been inhibited.

As the years and the illnesses progressed, Beryl retained her interest in engaging people and chatting with them. If I left her sitting while I went into a shop, she would invariably be exchanging ideas with the person sitting next to her when I returned.

I found myself, surprisingly, affected in a rather similar way. I became more inclined than I used to be to chat with taxi drivers and other people I came into contact with. I think this was because, as time went by, we came to have less and less chat at home. If I made a casual remark to Beryl about the television, or something we passed in the train or car, she would almost invariably not catch what I said, or not understand, or not be able to see what I was drawing her attention to. So I guess I gave up without quite realising it.

In some situations of confusion, or expression of disaffection, I was very surprised to hear a nurse say about Beryl, "It is the dementia speaking." I emphatically disagree – it was Beryl speaking, sometimes out of her frustration, although I do understand what the nurse means. And it is not always negative. We were enjoying a light lunch at a restaurant a while back, and both of us chatted to the waitress. We asked her name, and she said it was 'Chelsea'. Beryl said, "Very French!" Result – confusion all round, and some amusement.

It was around this time that I was surprised when one of the dementia nurses remarked that Beryl seemed 'old'. The nurse, with visits spaced of several weeks, was noticing deterioration that I was perhaps too close too see.

You're in charge

She would say repeatedly, "You're in charge", always with some irritation or even in a confrontational way. What she meant, I think, and what gave the force to her saying it was, "I'm not in charge (any longer)," in terms not of authority, but of capability. This was another of her portmanteau expressions of frustration.

It seemed that she had to wait, always wait, for me to do anything or everything. She had no option but to wait for me, for my timing, my inclination, my paying attention. I have been the one who is responsible, the decider, by default. A thoughtful, longstanding friend recently observed, "She was used to being in control." One day, recently, she was complaining about feeling old and tired. When I said I was too, she retorted, "You have more options." And when I was rushing around one day trying to get lots of jobs done, and obviously sounding rather fraught, she said, "Poor old you." As in some other rather sober situations, the latter remark was made, if not with a smile, at least with a half acknowledgement of being 'dramatic' in the not entirely serious sense. On another occasion, she said, in the same sort of way, "Oh dear, life and death!"

"Wherever we go, whatever we do, you are the one in charge," she said once. How I wished that was not the case. I have always been very happy being a car passenger rather than the driver, and often I have felt that I really would like someone else to arrange my day, and entertain me.

Health professionals tended to say and imply something that sounded similar, but in reality was very different. They said to me, "It is all up to you". There was some help to be had from medication, in calming agitation and improving sleep, but those effects were not reliable or consistent. So it came down, again, to me making the decisions about her clothes, her food, her entertainment, sometimes in the face of her questions or objections.

It was all up to me. Again, how I wish it were not.

11

"I'm sorry I'm not coping."
"Well you have to."

I'm sorry I'm not coping

It was a Sunday in early 2015. In the morning, I had taken Beryl to the local church where the anthem was from the Song of Songs, "Many waters cannot quench love", and one of the readings included the words, "If we love one another, God lives in us." I thought that was about enough challenges for one day, but I was encouraged and stimulated by joining in a few well-sung hymns. At home afterwards, she was restless, and complained, "You're so unhelpful, you don't pay attention at all." I am aware that sometimes I switch off. The challenge is frequently whether to engage or to ignore.

So the day went on, dragged on, with complaints about being tired and worn out; she was complaining, and I was echoing it back. I had had perhaps two or three hours of uninterrupted sleep the previous night, and she had had less. Furthermore, she had been into bed and out again probably twenty times during the day, with an average duration of stay in bed less than two minutes, and also she had been up and down the stairs a dozen times. As I tried to make a light supper for her, my voice was rather hoarse from frustration and stress (and probably from shouting too) when I said to her, "I should be able to cope better than this, but I'm sorry I'm not coping." Her response was, "Well, you have to." It was not said harshly or judgementally. It seemed just a bald statement of fact, and a reasonable one at that.

Less than half an hour later, I was struggling in the bathroom fitting her incontinence pads, with sweat running onto my glasses and into my eyes. While I was starting the whole exercise for a second time with one item broken and discarded, she looked at me. With, it seemed, half a grin she said, "I love you."

Occasionally in the evening, as she went to bed, I would kneel and talk to her quietly, and apologise for my weariness, and try to encourage her – one day at a time. That was not always very encouraging to me, let alone her.

This is part of what I have come to think of as 'extreme caring'. I have taken this idea from extreme sports and other extreme human activities. All are feats of endurance, and there are just as many ups and downs in the caring as in the sports, perhaps even more.

By extreme, I also mean that it may be unsustainable, and there are potentially even more profound challenges when 'extreme' takes on meanings such as approaching the end.

Burnout and meaning

During the five years before Beryl's stroke, I had occasion to think and read about what is called "burnout". Certainly, as the years went by after the stroke, I became exhausted as well as frustrated. Initially, in the immediate aftermath of Beryl's stroke, I offered to resign from my employment and from the various professional responsibilities that I had. I was impressed and surprised about how helpful and understanding all my groups of colleagues were. I managed to carry on with full-time work for six months, and in my professional responsibilities for a longer time. But roles at home and in the family changed immediately.

We met another couple in similar circumstances. The husband said clearly that he was an accountant and not a nurse. For me, perhaps by personality as well as training, the idea of being a carer seemed more natural or acceptable. I emphasise that this was a matter of inclination, not of virtue or moral superiority. In particular, as I managed with some part-time work, I felt that I learnt a little about being a working mother or a lone parent. I remembered Beryl's own experience with her newborn first baby, with no relatives in the country except me, and with me working hard and long in surgical training. She cared single-handed, even alone, for much of the time, and over the next few years her caring was demanding for her, sometimes debilitating.

The costs for me, and for us, after Beryl's stroke were considerable in every way, including finances such as loss of salary and pension. For the first time we needed to employ help around the house. That continued, and increased, for fifteen years. I learnt to be willing to accept help.

Burnout is often viewed as being related to stress, but in a situation such as ours stress seems to be quite inescapable. I remember being mildly surprised, but pleased, to be invited a long time ago to speak to a group of business people about stress. They were quite taken with one particular piece of research that I told them about, from an area of life far removed from theirs. In a study from the USA, complications in and after pregnancy were increased overall in women who had stressful life circumstances. But, whatever the level of stress, women with high levels of support during and after pregnancy were almost completely protected from having increased complications.[41] So support is vital, and it can come in a variety of forms. We have had great support from family and friends, and have adequate resources to support us too. But there is more to burnout than stress and support.

A particularly relevant book that I found was called *Beyond Burnout*[42]. A study of young professionals in public service roles found that burnout was associated with a loss of meaning, value or purpose in their work; with disillusionment, especially with the lack of a shared sense of values, or a shared quest for value. In the following chapters, I describe where Beryl and I have looked for and found meaning, and it is reassuring to read in numerous sources that even the *search* for meaning may provide support, especially if it is a collaborative search.

So full-time care meant that I was a carer all the time. The situation did not feel like the proverbial pressure cooker, but the pressure did certainly build up from time to time. It became increasingly difficult for me to leave Beryl by herself for any time at all. It began to seem that further measures were necessary.

Losing it completely

Picture this. Driving to visit our daughter and her family: me, the proponent of compassion and calm; and Beryl, on a familiar route normally taking about three hours plus stops. This particular day, the traffic everywhere is heavy and slow, and the journey will clearly take longer than usual. She starts saying, "Where are we going? Is this the right way? Will there be anyone there?" This is routine stuff, and I often cope with her repeating this sort of thing five times in ten minutes. But, because of the traffic, or because of something, she carries on. I try to drive steadily on the busy motorway, and I do, but the repeats go from five times in ten minutes to twenty times in half an hour to what seems like fifty times in fifty minutes. And I lose it completely – I explode. It feels as though my hair is standing on end, and I end up shouting and shouting for her to stop, including shouting "Shut up" which I cannot remember ever saying to her before in fifty years. I become alarmed that my voice is becoming hoarse, and then I feel appalled and extremely guilty. She opines from time to time that other people have "lost the plot", and often this seems to apply to her, but now I am the one who has lost it, completely. We manage to calm down and continue, me in contrite silence. Later, the penny drops. I am the one who is raging against the dying of the light.[43] It occurs to me that it is like some odd sort of road-rage, in-car rage, but that seems incidental.

Both of us had continuing losses. We lost conversations, between ourselves and with others. We lost friendships, at least with the depth and content that we used to have. Even good friends often talked over her or ignored her, as I did too when we were with friends. She had lost what? Everything? Not quite, not yet. The thought was worrying, dismaying.

Day care

Soon after Beryl's assessment at the Memory Clinic, we began to receive helpful input and advice during visits from social workers and nurses from the local council and NHS. One suggestion was about using local day centres as a break for me, and also a change for Beryl.

Over approximately two years, Beryl spent about two mornings or short days at two different day centres. The staff were all very competent and friendly, but Beryl did not find it easy to be with people with disabilities. This had become apparent in the early months after her stroke, when she did not enjoy a workshop in London about the use of computers for stroke sufferers.

Beryl was always an observer of people, and very sociable. And, at each of the day centres and care homes she was involved with, she had a reputation for trying to help, and for being solicitous of other clients or residents. She always, for example, complimented one *old gentleman* on his tie. She told me occasionally that some of the *children* (that's what she sometimes called the residents) were *helpless*. She said, "They don't know what to do. Some of those children are quite stupid." But she also said, "Some of the children are not very well." In later years, she even said, "Some of those people are dead." One particular woman at a day centre apparently used to talk constantly about herself and her family, including the importance of her deceased husband's job. With disarming insight Beryl said, "She says 'What are we doing next?' even more than I do." But a problem about socialising with other clients was always that her speech was jumbled by the dysphasia from the stroke (rather than from the dementia), and her good intentions were sometimes either not understood or even rebuffed.

The varied activities at the day centres included art and handicraft, which had never been a strong point for either Beryl or myself in terms of execution. But she enjoyed watching and trying. We were touched to see the simple still life in the photograph produced by a frail lady of about 80. She produced the piece during a session at the day centre, and we bought it for our kitchen wall. The funds went to the day centre, and the lady was delighted. "I've never sold a painting before," she said. A few weeks later, I saw she was not at the day centre session, and I was told that she had died.

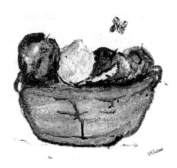

A simple still life in acrylics painted by a client at one of the day centres that Beryl attended

The second day centre Beryl went to was linked to a care home, and a few of the residents came to join in the activities. Beryl became aware of their presence, and it contributed to her gradually increasing resistance to going.

One day, driving home after leaving Beryl at the day centre, I felt that I would like to drop in to chat with a friend. The words that came to my mind were that I would like to have "some human contact". I wondered to myself what I meant – was she not human? It is the chat, the conversation, the exchange, that I think I had in mind; the everyday things, not focused on me and her and the caring.

The fact that I had to drive for one-and-a-half hours in total to have about two hours by myself meant that I looked for alternatives. But the idea of day centres linked to care homes had drawn my attention.

In late 2014, I opted for care and companionship for Beryl at home for one or two mornings each week, rather than at a day centre. We had used the service over the past year for occasional sitting with Beryl in the evening, when I was at rehearsals for choir or orchestra. The young woman who came from the service to be with Beryl, and sometimes take her out, was the one Beryl described as *affable*.

Respite and care

One of the jargon words that one comes upon quickly in the long-term care sector is *respite*. As jargon goes, it seems one of the better words. Long-term carers need a break, and it is a very good thing that public services acknowledge this. Although a break of even an hour or two is beneficial, respite of a week or two is really worth having if it is feasible. As some of our advisors said, it is hardly ever ideal for the one being cared for, but respite is of great importance for the carer to be able to carry on.

In the years after the stroke, before confusion set in, Beryl would often spend a day, or sometimes a weekend, with some of our family. The first time that "respite" really registered, as such (connected with "retreat"), was when old friends in London suggested that they would look after Beryl for a few days. I had a few quiet days at a retreat centre from the twelfth century, within walking distance of Canary Wharf in London.

Over the last five years, I was supported by those friends, and especially by our family, in taking breaks of a few days or a week; for example to get to Paris, or to a Benedictine Abbey on the Isle of Wight, or perhaps a Benedictine Convent in Leicestershire.

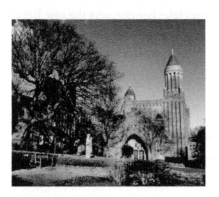

Quarr Abbey near Fishbourne, Isle of Wight, a quiet place for retreat and respite

Those were times of rest for me, of recharging my batteries, and also of exploration and discovery. I walked through Père Lachaise Cemetery and saw the tomb of Champollion, who deciphered the Rosetta stone.[44] This made me think of how I have to translate and interpret what Beryl says. I read a revelatory book[45] about the story of Job, which had some comfort to give in the face of distress and mortality. Overall, these times gave me an opportunity to reflect on our situation and scribble notes for this book, as well as physical exercise and emotional rest.

All these arrangements cost money; a lot more than everyday living. I remember my first time reading *The Doctor's Dilemma* by George Bernard Shaw,[46] when I was a medical student. The Preface was a penetrating view of medicine and health, and the memory was revived when I became involved in London in the 1970s in what was called 'social medicine'. In Shaw's view, what doctors needed to be able to prescribe was money and holidays. Even though aimed at underprivileged people in Victorian times, this principle also seemed relevant to our situation of needing respite.

Then one day, in December 2014, Beryl had her first episode of being unable to climb the stairs in our town house. We lived on three floors for twenty-five years, and going up the stairs was part of our exercise. But, on this occasion, she became breathless; she was, however, able to recover after a short rest. Nevertheless, on the next day, she subsided to the floor twice after climbing the stairs, and she was admitted to hospital. She was treated for pneumonia and recovered within two weeks. I helped her eat her traditional Christmas lunch in hospital.

In the month or two before she was admitted to hospital, there had been increasingly disturbed nights and early rising, and I had needed to make major rearrangements for changing beds and cleaning floors after accidents. So it was apparent that when Beryl came home from hospital, more changes would be needed.

While she was in the hospital, I managed to get a stair lift installed with remarkable speed. I moved to a separate bedroom to try to decrease the sleep deprivation, which was affecting both of us. I arranged for a care worker to come most mornings to help with bathing and dressing, which meant that I was not worn out by 9 o'clock each morning. In addition, through the initiative of family and friends, I was able to have one night most weeks away from the house altogether.

Respite for me again came into the conversation with professionals, as well as family and friends. We went back to two days a week at a day centre, in addition to the other support that I have just described. The day centre was in a different care home; our experience of care homes was expanding.

I am weary and I wish …

I have acknowledged my inability, or unwillingness, in the early months after the stroke to answer an unexpected question about what I was going to do when Beryl died. But, to be truthful, ideas of dying, cessation, ending, came to mind repeatedly over the duration, both early and late in the fifteen years of the process.

Walking along the Staffordshire and Worcestershire Canal a few years after the stroke, Beryl was desperately sad and depressed (I use the word in a clinical sense) about her incapacity and her loss. What came to my mind was the bottle of diazepam on the bedside at home. Would there be enough tablets to end it all? Probably. But this was her, and perhaps me, possibly wishing that she was dead, not that I was dead.

I remembered Tennyson's poem *Mariana*, about a young woman waiting for her lover. Beryl never enthused to me about Tennyson, and I would not have reciprocated. But he has many memorable lines, and I especially remember Mariana's refrain:

She said, I am aweary, aweary,
I would that I were dead!

Mariana also said, *My life is dreary, The night is dreary, The day is dreary, I am very dreary.* Mariana seems to have been altogether a dreary character, albeit constrained by the social customs of her day, as well as by the verse. Nonetheless, the refrain is what has stuck in my memory for many years, and it has seemed from time to time a reasonable summary of how Beryl, or I, or both of us felt. *I am aweary, aweary, I would that I were dead.*

Beryl has talked, from time to time, about being dead. Is it helpful or unhelpful – or perhaps disloyal – to remember that she said that sort of thing occasionally over the past forty-five years? She remembered a twenty-three-year-old British rugby player, paralysed in a training session and determined to end his life. He went to Switzerland after having attempted suicide at home three times, and she quite spontaneously expressed sympathy, understanding, perhaps fellow feeling.

Many people know at least some of what Thomas Hobbes wrote in *Leviathan*. If men lived without security there was, he wrote, "no society ... and the life of man, solitary, poor, nasty, brutish, and short."[47] I found myself remembering, with some embarrassment, that junior doctors used to talk sometimes about treating some old people as being like 'veterinary medicine'. And I found myself thinking that whatever else life was like at present, it did not seem short.

Beryl and I had little experience of death; my experiences in my clinical work somehow do not seem relevant in this context. Our four parents died since we were married, and on all four occasions we were in a different country. With the agreement of our families, we did not attend the funerals. The only family funerals that I have attended have been my two maternal grandparents, and Beryl's favourite aunt, who died from a massive stroke a few weeks before our wedding, while Beryl was still in Western Australia; a morbid antecedent.

We have not overall been morbid, however, and we have not discussed death at length, although some of the times when she talked about going *home*, even in the rehabilitation unit, I think she may have been obliquely referring to dying. A few years after the stroke, Beryl did ask a clergyman friend, to his surprise, if he would take her funeral. In addition, in tidying up her papers I found some notes from six months before the stroke. As part of her spiritual direction training, she completed some pages about "personal death awareness":

> *The death I would least prefer for myself would be:* a long awaited death at the end of a period of illness and disablement during which I had been a burden of care to my family and others
>
> *Self-written obituary:* died at age 80, suffered a heart attack; best remembered for challenging accepted ideas, rocking the boat, liberating people from things put upon them

I began looking at her papers when I started writing this book. By the time I found many items that were of relevance to our situation, she was not able to read or discuss any of them. So we never discussed this personal death awareness statement.

The unkindest cut

It is a long, hard task to be a carer, more so by definition if you are a full-time carer. And it can be a thankless task. However, neither I, nor any other carer whom I know, really look for thanks. In day-to-day life, adults who live together do not, I think, say "Thank you" to each other very many times in a day; much is taken for granted, and reasonably so.

So when, as part of our morning routine, I used to remove Beryl's non-slip shoes after helping her out of the bath, I was always slightly surprised when she almost always said, "Thank you". Similarly, if she said "Thank you" at other times, I was always slightly surprised. I think I can honestly say it very rarely, if ever, occurred to me that what might have been considered an appropriate expression of thanks had been omitted.

The most unkind cut of all, according to Mark Antony's speech in the aftermath of the assassination of Julius Caesar in Shakespeare's play, was "ingratitude". But I do not think that carers expect "gratitude" any more than thanks, or they certainly do not dwell on it even if it comes to mind. To me, "gratitude" easily links with "grovel", and carers do not wish to say or do anything that gives prominence to dependence rather than independence. As for Caesar, I can imagine that, Mark Antony notwithstanding, he might have preferred loyalty to gratitude.

But some remarks, and some behaviour, can fairly be perceived as cutting, there is no denying that. Waiting often seems unavoidable, both in day-to-day and in special situations, for example while tidying up, or preparing food, activities or outings. And, when it is suggested that the carer is just doing what they feel like or want to do, rather than getting on with the important activities, that can be wounding. The unkindest form of words in my experience was when she said, in the middle of one of our activities or negotiations, "Oh, it's all about you." There did not seem to be any calm or useful response to that expression, but it cropped up from time to time, in a slight variation of the words but with the same thought.

Again, the fundamental problem seemed to be frustration. While I may, sometimes, have had fits of self-absorption, I was never lazy any more than she was. I certainly had some different methods and time frames for organising, and this was often what provoked her outbursts. In addition, there was the somewhat paradoxical but common problem in illnesses such as Beryl's: the sufferer loses more and more of what we consider to be 'normal' self-awareness, but at the same time the sufferer seems to become more and more self-absorbed. The horizons narrow, and the walls close in. I remember being astonished when a friend remarked that there might be some comfort in the walls closing in; that could not have been further from my own experience.

Relentless

The word 'relentless' was often in my own thoughts, especially about our situation over the last year or two. I was pleasantly surprised when a visitor, who rarely saw Beryl, said, after observing the interactions within our home for a day or two, "Stuart, it is relentless." There was a sense, to which I have referred, that Beryl was commendably persevering. But there was also an overwhelming sense that the problems we faced daily were never solved; they were always there. The challenges, both physical and psychological, for both of us, went on relentlessly.

People talk about 'unrelenting love' as being important in the care of children, and we all agree. It applies in all aspects of caring but to me, in distinction perhaps from 'unconditional' love, it implies, or perhaps even confirms, that the problems are relentless.

Extreme caring

At the beginning of this chapter, I introduced my idea of extreme caring. It is a matter of ideas, but it is also a matter of feelings. Sometimes, I feel in myself, and I hear in others, what John Henry Newman called "cold dismay". I have recently had the moving experience of singing in Elgar's *Dream of Gerontius,* in which the words are part of his chilling description of the events in the garden of Gethsemane.[48] "Cold dismay" seems appropriate there, and it is hardly surprising that the words ring true to me. I have felt this cold dismay in sensing Beryl's feelings of abandonment. This feeling came out on many of the times I left her, but she also expressed it often when I was there with her.

Beryl has been one of many millions of sufferers, or clients, or patients, and likewise I have been one of many millions of carers. As a wise spokesperson for the German government said on television, in the immediate aftermath of the aeroplane crash into the French Alps in early 2015, "The sorrow is immeasurable." As for many profound ideas and sayings, these words go back to ancient Indian and Asian sources, and to the classical Greek dramatists.[49]

Often the loss that causes sorrow is sudden, and the grief wells up rapidly. But one of the aspects of extreme caring, as I describe it, is that it is a matter of endurance for all involved. The loss is slow and painful, and the grief ebbs and flows, but it becomes ever deeper. Any comparisons are unnecessary and unhelpful. As well as in the classics, there are profound insights in modern dramatists, even in unlikely places. As a diversion, I sometimes watch the frequently odd and melodramatic TV series set in the White House entitled *Scandal*. Recently, two bereaved characters ended up arguing about the magnitude of their losses.

The response was, "A broken heart is a broken heart; to take a measure is cruelty."

This sense of perspective – of large numbers affected, and of measureless sorrow – seems of great importance, but I must say that it is no consolation. Extreme caring is testing to the extreme.

12

"The people in that place had no idea of life, the universe, or ..."

From day centres to care homes

In late 2012, I received an invitation by mail to go to a special anniversary reunion with my medical school colleagues in Sydney, to be held in March 2013. I put it aside, feeling that it was just not feasible. The long-haul flights on our last visit to Australia, for Christmas 2011, had not been satisfactory, despite the fact that Beryl had enjoyed the same journeys many times since the stroke. And I did not think that she was well enough to manage the journey, or enjoy several weeks in Australia. However, to my astonishment, she came across the letter of invitation, picked it up, understood at least the general drift of its contents and said, entirely spontaneously, "You must go. I will stay somewhere."

So I went, having investigated local care homes with our family and decided on a small place about twenty minutes from home. This was Beryl's first experience of staying in a residential care home, rather than just going for day care. She was there for nineteen nights while I squeezed in a two-week visit to Australia. I had arranged visitors for Beryl every day, including some outings. It was not a success. She hated it.

That was the place that she described as *torpid*, which seemed a fair comment. The staff were kind and helpful, the managers especially so. But Beryl's comments were, "When you were away I was on my own. Nobody cares, nobody loves me. It was – they were – horrible."

That was the place about which she said, "The people in that place had no idea of life, the universe or ... " (the sentence tailed off). The family had picked up that saying from Douglas Adams's book in the 1980s.[50] About that place, and repeatedly and frequently afterwards, whether at other care homes or day centres, or in our own home, she would say, "People wouldn't talk to me," and "People laugh at me." Once, her comment was, "They all said, 'Ha ha ha, silly old person'."

I understood how the few residents in that care home who were capable of having a conversation might have given up trying to talk with her, because of the muddled language of her dysphasia. But her complaint about people laughing at her was more difficult to gauge. I knew that sometimes Beryl said to the family, and to other people, "Happy birthday" as a general greeting, especially as a toast with a glass of fizz. And it seemed possible that some people in the care homes might have laughed with amusement, as family and friends often did, with good humour. But I wondered if sometimes she was delusional and hallucinating, which can be part of some dementia experiences. At a day centre, some time later, she said she that could see a laughing face behind her chair; at least, I think that what was she said. She was started on a new drug soon after that, but she continued to comment about people laughing at her.

That first period of respite care in a care home was followed by several other periods. Just a few months after I returned from that reunion in Australia, I was due to go to Normandy in France for a weekend, singing with a local choir. I visited and chose quite a different sort of care home in the New Forest. It turned out that I needed to go to London for the long weekend instead of France, and it was just as well. The family took Beryl to the care home, but she decided that she did not want to stay, so she ended up with the family for a few days. I would have been very distressed if I had not been easily contactable. The family coped brilliantly, as always, but I was conscious that neither Beryl nor I was dealing with the respite "system" very well.

A year later, I had another singing expedition, this time a week involving Spanish renaissance music in Santiago de Compostela. Nurses and care workers who were supporting us and advising me at home had emphasised that residential respite care was never really going to be greeted enthusiastically by the one being cared for. So I made arrangements with an organisation that provided full-time care in the client's own home. It seemed to me that this approach would map much more onto Beryl's wishes, and have a reassuring familiarity. I had a really enjoyable and uplifting time away, but returned to find major dramas. We had arranged for Beryl to have the first few days with our local family and, in retrospect, that arrangement had added to the disruption. The few days with the live-in carer were very stressful for all, with Beryl wanting to visit family all the time, and complaining about the carer. It had seemed like a good idea at the time, but it misfired.

Three months later, I was continuing to feel the strain. Writing this makes me feel that I really was not coping very well; I needed another break already. In consultation with the family, I chose yet another care home, close to family and friends, and again arranged daily visits for Beryl. Then I went off to Paris again for a week by myself. I returned to find Beryl dismally clutching some of her books and looking rather bedraggled, waiting for me. It was a very caring care home, but friends thought that Beryl was more challenging for them to look after than everyone had expected. Again, Beryl was very uncomfortable being with people who were very disabled mentally or physically.

Fading – and the fading of the light

At home, Beryl continued to spend less time looking at books, and became less interested in music with words, preferring instrumental music. But at the same time she began more and more to carry books around the house with her, and to want to take them out to the day centre, or simply in the car. They were books of words, especially Jim Cotter, but also art books and books of our own photographs. It was as though that was one way of her keeping in touch with the content – words and pictures – and with the memories and the meanings contained in those pages.

She was fading; the light was fading. I have talked about 'losing it completely' in a general, colloquial way, and in that context I alluded to Dylan Thomas, and raging against the dying of the light. But it was the word and the idea of 'fading' that stayed with me. Perhaps I wanted to avoid using the word, even the idea, of 'dying' if I could.

Quakers talk about 'holding people in the light', and this means a lot to me. I wondered if somehow I, and Beryl, might be able to share the light that we had, so that there might be some compensation for the fading.

I found some consolation in the words of Elizabeth Barrett Browning, "when light is gone, love remains for shining." Those gentle words are in fact part of her poem *To*

Flush, My Dog,[51] and they refer to waiting rather than the death of human or dog. But the feelings and understandings are surely no less poignant. However, I held onto the fact that the light had not gone, yet.

Accepting help

I described, in the previous chapter, how I accepted more help at home once Beryl returned from hospital after Christmas 2014. But the questions about suitable care homes for respite and day care remained. Then, through an acquaintance at the local choral society, I learnt about a new purpose-built home within reasonable distance. I visited, and was impressed with the thoughtful design and the caring welcome for me. The home had only been open a matter of months, and there were not many residents. Beryl began immediately to go for two mornings each week, and established special relationships with several of the staff. She did not like noisy or disruptive residents, but there were few of those.

In March 2015, Beryl spent two weeks as a resident there, with frequent visits from family and friends, but not going out. My idea was that she would be comfortable with staff and facilities which she had come to know through the day care, and that worked out reasonably; certainly much better than the previous experiences with care homes.

All my advisers encouraged me to try to take a break three or four times a year. Of course, this was costly, in terms of money and also in a personal way with me leaving her, and her feeling left. But, after we had managed a short holiday with friends in the west of Scotland in June, I took another break in July while Beryl had two more weeks in the care home. She seemed more settled when I returned; contented may be too strong a word.

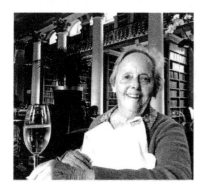

Beryl enjoying a champagne cream tea in the Signet Library in Edinburgh a month before admission to the care home

After that, we enjoyed a few days in Edinburgh in August 2015, seeing a special young friend of Beryl's. But she went missing when I was buying coffee while waiting for the return flight. I found her down the escalator outside the non-return doors of the departure lounge, looking for me, even though I had never been out of sight. And the more routine daily challenges were increasing, so in September, for the first time, I discussed full-time care with a new care home, in the same organisation but nearer to our house.

The things Beryl said during the month from August to September 2015 emphasise where she was in her thoughts and feelings. "I'm old and fragile," she said. While in our own house, she said "Where are you? Where are they? I don't know where I am." To her frequent saying of "They all laugh at me," she added, extraordinarily, "They look at me as though I was a spaceship." And, frequently, also said "I'm so fed up, I can't go on." Those last words sound like me voicing my feelings, but it was in fact her.

Events moved rapidly. Beryl was admitted to the care home before the end of September 2015. Technically, she was admitted for one month's respite care, with the option of staying on. This was partly as a trial, and partly to give time to clarify financial support.

The worst thing

A month after the respite period in July 2015, Beryl said to me, "The worst thing in my mind is that you will be going away again." I did not respond. I did not know what to say. I knew that our situation was becoming ever more demanding, but what Beryl said stirred up in me not just fresh concerns, but also old memories.

I remember well an experience from fifty years ago that I have never discussed with anyone since then. Beryl's father, blinded in an accident twenty-five years before that, was becoming more and more disabled, and the family could no longer manage to care for him at home. They found a care home, and when it came to the day of his admission, I was the one designated, as a new son-in-law, to take him there. I was emotionally involved in quite a different way from the rest of the family, not least because of the relative shortness of the time I had known him. Also, he seemed to relate to me as a man differently from how he related to the three women in his life. In the event, we arrived at the home. I remember taking him into a sparse room; he was unable to see any of the details of the room. I spent just a matter of minutes explaining that this was it, and I left him. The way I felt meant that I could not avoid the word "abandon" in my mind. I do not, in any way, mean that I thought the family were abandoning him – they certainly did not. But Beryl and I never saw him again. We left Sydney for London very soon after, and he died within six months.

Abandonment

The feelings when I abandoned Beryl's father, for whom I had only a small and short-term share of responsibility, were magnified – almost overwhelming – when I took the plunge/ conceded defeat/gave in/took her away/sent her away. These were my confusions of thought then, and they persisted.

I can remember the feeling of unreality; going out the door of our house, thinking that Beryl would never return home again, and that she had no idea of what was happening. I think that was one of the very few times I have felt what might be called *guilt*, in the midst of all the other emotions.

When Beryl's sister's husband was admitted to a care home in Australia, because of increasingly aggressive dementia, she said, with great distress, that it was *cruel*. That summarised the whole situation: the illness itself, the environment, the necessity of leaving him in confusion and distress. It seemed to me an honest and true assessment, not just of feelings but also of the reality. I understood just what she meant.

I remembered that Beryl wrote, before her stroke, that she did not want to be a burden because of illness and disablement. I hoped that I might be right in feeling that was some sort of permission or acceptance of us "handing over" her practical care to others.

Conceding defeat

I then began the early stages of experiencing what Beryl's sister and many thousands of other carers knew. Even if someone else carried on with the day-to-day caring, the caring by me did not stop. It became different, in some ways even more challenging. There was the possibility of more time and energy to carry on. For example, when my sleep was disturbed it was by the restlessness of my own heart and mind, rather than by someone else's restlessness. But the coming and going of visiting was very wearing, and the feeling of frustration at not being able to cope, or to ameliorate some of the problems, did not diminish.

More often than not, when I visited, Beryl wanted to come home. Sometimes this was expressed very tearfully, sometimes in irritation and anger. This was the aspect of her being in a care home which I had most dreaded, and the fact that it seemed to be a common experience was no consolation. No doubt my feelings of heartbreak arose from the fact that I still cared.

Long term care

It was in September 2015 that Beryl moved into long-term care. I felt myself setting out on a journey of entirely unknown length and complexity. Part of the uncertainty was financial. The payments required were very large indeed, even if some support from local government was possible, conditional on our personal finances being arranged appropriately. Beryl had had no personal income for twenty-five years, so some help seemed possible and did in fact transpire.

Arranging finances was just one my many new responsibilities. I had to learn about entirely new dimensions of health and social care, and to deal with government departments that I did not previously know existed.

But all these details of length and complexity passed Beryl by. I think she felt that she was back in respite care, although she would not have known the word. The only difference, to begin with, was that I visited every day instead of not appearing at all for two weeks or more.

When we arrived at the care home for her admission, she was welcomed by several members of staff, each of whom extended their left hand to her to shake hands. This was an impressive beginning. They had all been told of – and remembered and acted upon – the fact that Beryl's right hand and arm had not functioned normally since the stroke, and that she tended to reach out with her left hand.

It was a quiet place, newly purpose-built and opened just a few months prior with, as yet, only a small number of residents. I had been able to take some steps in personalising her room, with numerous paintings and embroidery from home, and some of her own furniture. She had many of her own favourite books, DVDs and CDs. She learnt quickly to see her name on the door of her room.

In the first few days, we watched many music DVDs, and enjoyed a garden party in the sunny grounds of the home, which was by the water only three miles from our house. Beryl was restless, as she had been at home, and she tended to pace the corridors when I was not there.

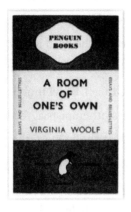

A large mounted reproduction of this book cover was one of the art works which I put on the wall to help make it feel like Beryl's own room.

Beryl's period of settling in was abruptly interrupted when on the tenth night she fell while pacing the corridors at 10pm. She had not wanted to go to bed. I arrived after half an hour to be with her and to help the night staff, but she lay in a pool of blood on the floor for nearly four hours before an ambulance was able to get to her. She had gashed her head, and her left arm was obviously uncomfortable.

At the hospital, she was seen in the same Emergency Department as for the stroke fifteen years before; the department where I had been an honorary consultant thirty-five years ago. She was assessed and X-rayed rapidly, and her cut head stitched. The staff expressed concern about her head injury, and she was transferred to a ward, near where she had been ten months previously with pneumonia. I was rather irritated by the fact that I had to harass the doctors and persuade them to carry out the X-ray of her left shoulder that revealed a fracture. The problem had, in fact, been noticed in the Emergency Department, but they had allowed themselves to be distracted by the head injury. Fortunately, no intervention was needed with the fracture, and the whole admission was taken up with trying to get Beryl mobile enough to return to the care home. The physiotherapists agreed that she would regain mobility better back at the home rather than in hospital. However, the doctors insisted on her staying in hospital over the next weekend because of a non-specific abnormal blood test. As I expected, Beryl had no help at all with mobility over the weekend. I write all this detail down because it stuck in my mind. It is not so much an adverse criticism or a complaint as it is recognition of how complex and demanding it is to care for older people, especially those with dementia as well as other disabilities.

Beryl's mobility never returned to what it had been. She was able walk a little around the care home with help, and I took her out to garden centres or shopping malls in her wheelchair.

The other residents, and their families, were pleasant, and not noisy. But some were very confused, and Beryl did not like them coming into her room. Within three months, two of the residents had died, one who had entered the home after Beryl. This, again, is not a criticism, but a reflection on the sort of problems that type of care entails. It seemed very different for those residents who needed care because they had been living by themselves, rather than because of mental deterioration.

There were many activities in the care home, and Beryl joined in most. The staff attempted to create some sort of community, and they had quite reasonable success. I went to some of the music and quiz groups with her. She enjoyed visits by children from local nurseries. We had looked forward to what was advertised as a Happy Hour. That never worked well, partly for practical reasons, but I cannot resist repeating the remark in an episode of the Simpsons where Homer is told to lighten up: "You're making Happy Hour bitterly ironic."

She had visitors from time to time, and she smiled especially whenever the grandchildren came. But she had repeated chest infections, and her mobility continued to decrease. She would walk little, often clutching her books that she would scarcely look at, but still hold tight to her. She was often distressed, and would call out or shout.

I took the occasional day off from visiting; our son was especially committed to visiting, and his family frequently visited too. But I was conscious that, in a way I had not anticipated, I still felt entirely responsible for her. I had handed over the physical caring, and the nights, and most of the day care too. And I never felt responsible for her illnesses, or her confusion or unhappiness. But I retained this inescapable feeling that somehow I was responsible for trying to keep her happy. Yet I am, of course, conscious that for much of the time I was not there anyway.

Some visits were easier than others. Sometimes we could do things together. Sometimes she just wanted to rest. One memory that still reverberates is of a day when I left after a short-ish visit, when she had been rather fractious. "Don't run away," she said to me in a loud and distressed voice. Even now, I feel bad to remember that. It is hard not to concede that this memory is one of the few that fall into the 'guilty' category.

After three months in the care home, I joined in Christmas lunch with most of the other residents and one or two family members. It was a very good meal, but Beryl did not enjoy it. Most noticeably, she did not enjoy the champagne that I had taken for us and any other residents. That was a sign that she really was not doing very well.

Contented – or not?

At the end of his moving book subtitled *How dementia stole the love of my life*,[52] John Suchet tells of his discussion with the staff of the care home to which his wife was admitted. They said that such places, and their residents, could be quite contented.

It is true that people with advanced dementia may become withdrawn and silent. I have already related how Beryl described the first care home in which she stayed as *torpid*. But another home to which she went for day care and respite had more than one noisy and aggressive resident.

Beryl herself did not settle in the care home where she had become a long term resident. She was occasionally noisy, holding her head and calling out with frustration. She was not content. In many ways, she experienced that *lost content* of the Shropshire Lad. She wanted to go back to the old days, where her remembered abilities and achievements obviously outweighed her memories of challenges, difficulties and unhappiness.

I said to myself, and to friends, that I did not expect her ever to settle in the care home. If she were to become, or appear to be, content, I said I would feel as though in some ways I had completely lost the real Beryl with whom I had lived for fifty years. She was never really content, and it never occurred to me to tell her that she should be.

I think often of one of George Bernard Shaw's smart remarks: "The reasonable man adapts himself to the world: the unreasonable one persists in trying to adapt the world to himself. Therefore all progress depends on the unreasonable man."[53] For my own purposes, I interpret 'unreasonable' as meaning awkward or questioning rather than irrational. My modification of the saying, related to Beryl and others, is to suggest that the contented person goes along with the world as it is, whereas the uncontented person, the 'discontent', if you like, is the one who tries to change things, or at least wishes things were different.

So, in what might seem a rather perverse way, I wanted Beryl to go on – she needed to go on – and not to become content if that meant, as I felt it would, that she became, in her own good word, *torpid*.

Extreme care

After Christmas 2015 in the care home, Beryl became very immobile and resistant to moving. We managed few outings. She was quieter, but no less distressed. She did not seem to be able to throw off the chest infection that had grumbled along for weeks.

Our daughter visited with me on a Saturday morning in mid-January. Living 200 miles away, she did not get to see Beryl as often as she would have liked, and she noticed immediately that Beryl was not breathing easily. I guess that I would have realised it, but not as quickly as the fresh pair of eyes saw it. At our prompting, the staff called an ambulance, and reported some other chest problems to the paramedic who arrived quickly. Soon, there were four young men in the room, and Beryl was manoeuvred into the ambulance with some difficulty.

After that visit our daughter remarked that Beryl seemed perhaps to be beyond being comforted, which had always been one of my aims. Nevertheless, despite looking and feeling unwell, Beryl thanked the young student paramedic to whom she had been chatting, and smiled at this group of strapping young men.

In the hospital, we followed her from one assessment unit to another, and then to the ward. She was not easy to assess or manage. After the weekend, I spoke with staff about Beryl needing more nursing care in the care home. Everyone agreed; her decline had been more rapid than anyone expected. So, with considerable speedy support and understanding from the care home organisation, I was able to arrange for Beryl to be transferred, after discharge, to a different care home within the same organisation that had nursing facilities. Beryl was assessed by staff of the new care home while she was on the hospital ward. She seemed to be recovering, and I moved all her clothes, books and furniture from the original care home to the new place that was close to the rehabilitation unit in the New Forest, where Beryl had been after the stroke fifteen years previously.

All parties agreed that Beryl would remain in the hospital over the next weekend in order to have a full hospital discharge assessment on the Monday. But the hospital called me on the Saturday morning to say that Beryl was having problems with her breathing. By the time I reached the hospital, her breathing had stopped; she had died shortly before I arrived. I said my goodbyes, and as occupational therapy I spent the next few hours moving all Beryl's things back from the new care home to our house, while the family were travelling to be with me.

So this was care in the extreme, care to the extreme. With little notice, the care – at least the sort of care in which I had been engaged for so long – had come to an end.

Thinking about meaning

In one sense our story in this book is ended, in terms of telling it as it happened. Our struggle, separately and together, to find meaning in our lives took place while the story was unfolding, but I did not want to interrupt the narrative.

So readers may well find something of a change of tone in the next few chapters. There is at least as much of thinking as of feeling; of the head as of the heart. The meaning we have found for Beryl has been in the feelings much more than in any ideas. But for me the concepts have been fundamental, as I have lived with our progressing and deteriorating situation, and they continue to be so in my changed way of life.

The chapters about meaning in images and music, and in silence, were largely written before Beryl became resident in the care home. The final two chapters, about meaning in caring and about going on, have been modified by our experiences with residential care, and following Beryl's death.

Meaning in images

Rehabilitation

A few weeks after Beryl's stroke, while she was still in the rehabilitation unit, some therapy assistants came to see her to help with her speaking. They brought cards of words and pictures, such as in the illustration – rather basic and, I thought (maybe incorrectly), old-fashioned. Beryl was utterly unimpressed. As she said in the interview in 2005, "I can't see any cats and

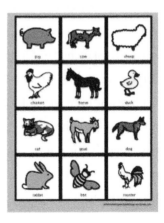

dogs and all that silly business." By "can't see", she meant that she did not want to see or discuss that sort of thing. The family did, however, produce a variety of scrapbooks with photographs of the family and of everyday objects. But Beryl was never very interested in them either.

Talking with pen and paper

The excellent speech and language therapist, who spent three years helping Beryl develop her conversation about topics and ideas that interested and motivated her, helpfully pointed out that Beryl was a very visual person. This neatly summarised what we knew – that Beryl loved books, holding them, and turning the pages, and certainly not listening to recorded books or talks which she had disliked long before the stroke.

One of the therapist's basic principles was that when with Beryl she always had a notepad and pen in her hand. She constantly sketched out something connected with what she and Beryl were saying; either a few actual words, or rough sketches of places or even ideas. I admired and accepted her approach, but I have to admit I was never very good at doing what she did. In the heat of the moment, it rarely, if ever, occurred to me to pick up pencil and paper.

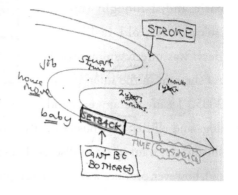

The way in which the therapist illustrated what they were talking about is shown in these two pictures. First, they were discussing problems in the early months after the stroke occurred, with changes of house and changes with my work and my time.

By the time we decided to move back to Southampton, the therapist had ceased to have any formal work involvement with Beryl

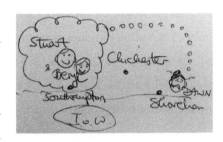

and had become a friend. In talking with Beryl, she illustrated in the second picture the changes in geography, but also the maintenance of connections in the second diagram.

A room with a view

Beryl grew up within view of the Pacific Ocean in Sydney, and always enjoyed being near the water. The house to which we retreated after Beryl's stroke backed onto a beach on the

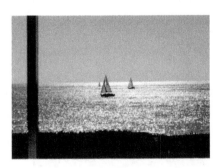

Beryl's sitting room in Rustington

English Channel, about twenty miles west of Brighton. By beach,

I mean a typical stony British beach rather than an Australian beach with golden sand, but Beryl had become acclimatised to the difference. The full windows and balcony on the first floor looked south across the channel.

Beryl would sit for hours looking out. It was quiet, with only a few sailing dinghies close to the shore in the summer, and occasional larger ships almost on the horizon. But there were wonderful sunsets; sunrises too, but we did not see many. And in the evening we could watch the wading birds, the striking colours of the oystercatchers, and the twinkle-toes of the beach, the sanderlings. Often we saw larger birds, especially crows, and also cormorants perched on the groynes or lampposts. The view was not always predictable. One day, to the astonishment of our neighbours who asked in jest if we were under attack, there was an eye-level flypast, only a few yards offshore, of a dozen small and medium-sized warplanes, old and new, in honour of an RAF retirement home almost next door to our house.

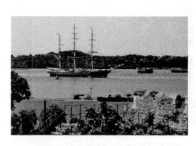

A tall ship on Southampton Water from Beryl's sitting room

Five years after the stroke, we moved to Southampton and were fortunate to find a house very similar to that in Rustington. Having three storeys gave us a good view of Southampton Water, with its great variety of cruise ships, cargo ships and sailing boats.

Beryl would sit for a long time and watch. She regularly waited for the standard 5pm sailing time of the cruise ships.

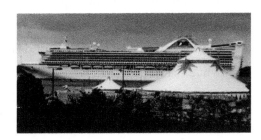

From our window: a cruise ship departing plus the bonus of the big top of the Moscow State Circus

The views from our sitting rooms were a major focus for all of the fifteen years that Beryl spent at home after the stroke. Getting up the flights of stairs to see the view was always a strong motive for her to keep mobile, starting from when she was initially in the rehabilitation unit.

We were fortunate in the location of our town house. Beryl never tired of her room with a view. In later years, she could still see the ships

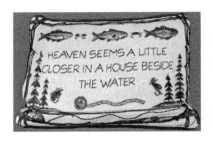

from her armchair without having to get up to sit in the chair in the bay window. I bought her a small cushion that whimsically summed up her attitude, and mine.

Art and life

As we began to be able to assemble our own collection of art, we started with still life and landscapes, and also what I am told are called genre paintings of everyday scenes that do not quite fit either still life or landscape. Then we developed further interest in more abstract paintings. Beryl had her own interests and made her own choices, some surprising. Certainly having a large number of paintings, large and small, around the house provided her with interest every day, and I think that qualifies as providing her with some sort of meaning.

Still life

As an example of what might, I suppose, be called real still life, Beryl was always drawn to the elaborate arrangements of candleholders in our local church. One of the first services that we attended there had all the candles lit. The photograph shows just some of the arrangement.

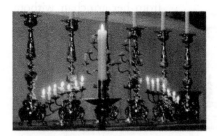

Candles at St Michael's Church, Southampton City Centre

Another still life, in terms of an artefact, that was of immense significance to Beryl was the medallion from a necklace that we bought from a Hopi artist in Arizona, ten years after Beryl's stroke. The Hopi Tribe are a peaceful nation, and

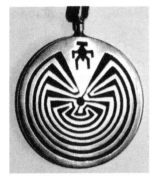

Beryl and I both perceived the design as reminiscent of traditional western labyrinths that have been very important for Beryl. The woman from whom we made the purchase said she had also suffered a stroke, which added to the meaning of the exchange and of the medallion.

Hopi medallion

Traditional still life painting was one of our interests for many years. This is one of several pieces we bought a few years before Beryl's stroke. We were interested in the artist as a woman from the Midlands, some years older than Beryl.

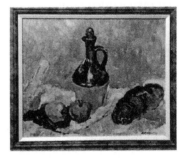

Beryl herself arranged the purchase of a large abstract still life for me about five years ago. She chose that particular piece because one of the few words that she could decipher in the

catalogue was 'burgundy', which is the red colour of the left side of the painting on the wall, and which she knew was my favourite wine.

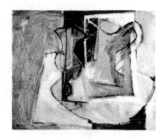

Burgundy pitcher

Landscapes live and painted, and everyday scenes

The first substantial painting that we bought was Beryl's choice, and it remained one of her favourites. It was always peaceful to look at, and as the years went by it connected with her enjoying our own garden room.

Beryl would sit and look at paintings like this, or walk past them, sometimes with a comment. They were part of her daily environment, amongst other things a visible connection to the past.

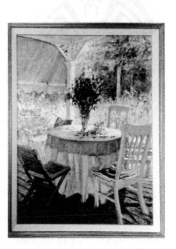

The first painting which Beryl purchased, a few years before her stroke, and which was a constant and peaceful companion

At two quite separate primary schools in Sydney in the 1940s, we each owned an ochre-coloured paperback book with the title *The Wide Brown Land*. It was an anthology of contemporary Australian poetry, the most famous poem being *My Country* by Dorothea Mackellar.[54] Many people, not just from growing up in Australia, might know the first line *I love a sunburnt country*. However, I learnt only recently that those words were the beginning of the second stanza, not the first. The first lines of the poem, which was written in England, address a British reader familiar with words and features like 'coppice', and with green and shaded lanes. The poem is all about how landscapes vary, and how hearts become attached to different landscapes.

Before we were married, Beryl visited the famous red monolith Uluru in central Australia, and also outback Western Australia. We both, at different times, crossed the Nullarbor Plain by train. In the years after the stroke, we visited Australia many times, often bringing back paintings reminiscent of a wide land which, if not always brown, was certainly rarely green and shaded. Beryl chose a small multimedia abstract triptych entitled *Torched, Scorched, and Burnt Land*.

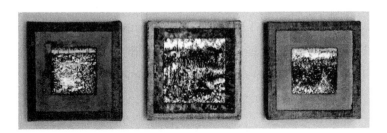

The three small paintings hung in our garden room and moved to Beryl's room in the care home. She was always looking at them; on the wall, the pictures are brown and black with small upper sections of light that, in the outer two, is a tiny touch of blue sky. The bushfire theme is clear.

A bright Australian landscape with gum trees (*eucalyptus* to the British) was what Beryl declared as her favourite as she was going into the care home. I hung it on the wall of her room there. It is a large bright painting that I brought back from the Southern Highlands, a little south of Sydney.

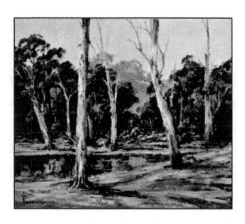

An Australian billabong

However, Beryl had lots of 'favourites', another being a European landscape; an open woods scene in the next illustration. That ended up on her wall in the care home also.

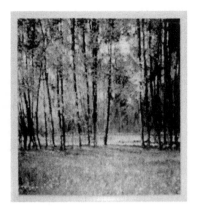

On Beryl's wall the painting was all gentle blue-grey and gold and green, over brown tree trunks

I am very aware that some of our family, and many of our friends, are more attached to the physical outdoors than we have ever been. This involves walking, and travelling, but it seems more than that. Some of them have a real affinity for the natural world, a love of natural landscapes. Peter Lanyon, one of the St Ives artists, said that landscape, the outside world of things and events larger than ourselves, is the proper place to find our deepest meanings.[55] Simon Schama wrote about trying to find in nature a consolation for our mortality.[56]

Despite the challenges, Beryl and I managed to explore and appreciate some aspects of landscape. We travelled across the United States by train and wondered at what we saw: an area the size of Australia with such variety and contrast. The photograph shows Beryl enjoying the central west.

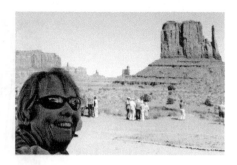

Beryl in Monument Valley, Arizona – taken inside a tour coach

We were fortunate in getting back to Venice, a place where seascape, landscape and portraits combine, just a short time before Beryl was hospitalised with pneumonia in December 2014, from which she never really recovered. Beryl loved the varied ambience of Venice. On a previous visit, we had stayed at a separate little island, where she enjoyed sitting in a quiet wooded garden, looking at her beloved Jim Cotter books with rabbits near her feet.

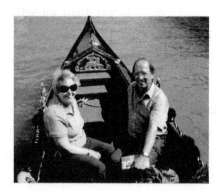

Beryl's treats in Venice – gondola rides, this from 2009

Galleries and portraits

In the year before Beryl's stroke, she was a steward at the Globe Theatre in London. We lived just around the corner, which meant that we were also near neighbours of the Tate Modern gallery. Just nine days before Beryl's stroke, as local residents, we were among the many guests at the official opening of Tate Modern by the Queen.

Those specific contacts were wiped out by the stroke, but we have been able to visit many galleries around the world. The travel and the galleries have maintained alertness and interest, for me as the carer as well as for her, and it has often involved a larger group than just two.

At the beginning of this book, I showed a photograph of Beryl in one of the many galleries we visited in Amsterdam over the years. We have another very similar photograph of her viewing Van Gogh's *Harvest with Blue Cart* in Amsterdam. The painting does not show very clearly, so I have shown just the painting here. Beryl often talked

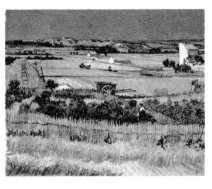

Van Gogh's Harvest with Blue Cart

about remembering the blue cart (in the centre of the painting) from her primary school days.[57]

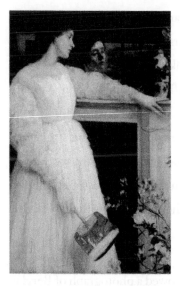

Symphony in White, No. 2: The Little White Girl, by James Abbott McNeill Whistler, 1864

Over the past twenty years, Beryl was very taken with portrait painting, especially by women artists, or involving women as subjects. A year or so before her stroke she was absorbed by the exhibition "On Reflection" at the National Gallery in London, curated by Jonathan Miller. We bought the book of the exhibition and Beryl would browse it often, including for many years after her stroke. The particular painting that attracted her was a study of a young woman in white by James McNeill Whistler. There was something of the pensiveness, the wistfulness perhaps, the reflectiveness, of that painting that drew her back again and again, including many times after her stroke.

Beryl was a Friend of the Royal Academy in London. She enjoyed frequent visits, latterly using a wheelchair. I have to admit that for the last year or two she enjoyed a long lunch and a short visit to the galleries, but including the train journey, which she enjoyed, it was always a pleasant and, I think, meaningful day out.

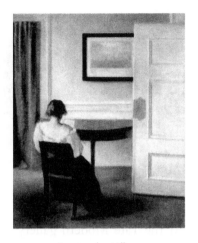

She particularly enjoyed the exhibition of the paintings of the Danish artist Vilhelm Hammershøi that was

Interior, by Villem Hammershøi, 1898

subtitled "the poetry of silence". This was eight years after her stroke. She looked with absorption at painting after painting of quiet interiors, with young women who were always looking away. We bought the catalogue, and for years she would leaf through it, never tiring of the variety and the sameness.

We were able, several times, to visit the Orangerie in Paris, built to accommodate Monet's enormous crescent-shaped paintings of water lilies. Beryl was especially pleased to have, occasionally, a room to herself, as the photograph shows.

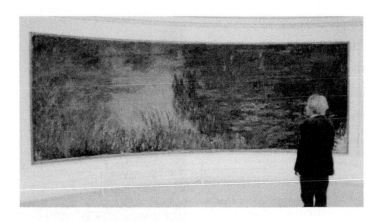

At the Tate Modern gallery in London, we saw one of the enormous metal spider sculptures by Louise Bourgeois. Beryl was diverted, as I was, to find other examples not only at the Museum of Modern Art in San Francisco, but also in the Scottish National Gallery of Modern Art in Edinburgh.

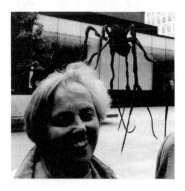

San Francisco Museum
of Modern Art

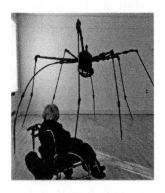

Scottish National
Gallery, Edinburgh

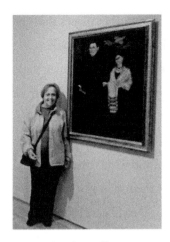

Beryl had a large collection of art books by and about women artists. Having discovered and enjoyed the National Museum of Women in the Arts in Washington, D.C., she then tracked down, with my help, paintings by Frida Kahlo in San Francisco.

Beryl with a self portrait of Frida Kahlo and her husband Diego Rivera at the Museum of Modern Art in San Francisco in 2010

Beryl's Life Story Book

As the years passed, and as Beryl's memory faded, I produced, at the suggestion of one of the nurses who came to support us at home, several photo books of family and holidays, including reminders of many of the gallery visits. In particular, I produced Beryl's Life Story Book using old and new images to remind Beryl and to inform new acquaintances.

The book, in several versions, covered the time from before Beryl went to school up to the present. The staff in the various day centres and care homes were delighted and impressed. These were portable pictures and Beryl carried them everywhere with her. She was pleased to sit and go through the books again and again, with new people or with people who had seen them lots of times. It included many of our travels, and Beryl was always pleased to talk about Australia, and about other places that she had been to which were illustrated in her life story book.

I am inclined to think that the suggestion to produce these books was among the most important things that the health or social services did for Beryl over the whole time of her illness. The deliberate use of images had also begun with our star speech and language therapist. I learnt much, and we all benefited from the advice and encouragement about the use of images that we had from her and all her successors in Beryl's care.

A room of one's own

When Beryl was admitted to the care home, my aim was to make her room seem as much like her own space as possible. The gum trees and woodland paintings, and the burnt land triptych, were all on her walls, together with another favourite which was also very popular with visitors at home, as well as in the care home.

This was a small painting of a slightly abstract seaside scene. Beryl loved the combination of seaside and young people.

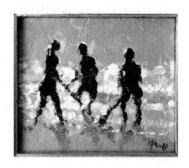

On prominent display were several of Beryl's own tapestries.

Beachcombers

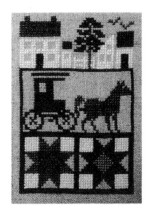

Amish country
embroidered by Beryl

At home, an embroidered bell-pull had hung on the landing for many years. Over the past few years, Beryl would remark, every time she walked past, "I did that!" I have illustrated here a charming small embroidery that Beryl made following a visit to Amish country with friends a year or two before her stroke. It was hung in Beryl's room for many years.

Beryl also liked to have icons and crosses on the wall. We had not grown up in that tradition at all, but as words faded, it seemed that those images came to be important to her.

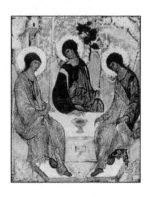

A small reproduction of the Rublev icon was in Beryl's room

Before her stroke, Beryl had become aware of the albatross flying close to the waves as a picture of life's challenges, and this view was reinforced after the stroke. She would sometimes listen to a recording of TS Eliot himself reading his Four Quartets. She chose, with my help, words from the end of East Coker[58] to summarise some of her thoughts and feelings a few years after the stroke; the ideas were of the waves and the wind and the darkness and the desolation – and of a bird flying over the water.

The care home where she became a resident was beside the water, and all the communal spaces had seaside-themed names. Just outside Beryl's room, in the corridor, was a space called Crow's Nest, with a photograph of an albatross. As Beryl's awareness faded, the albatross was a constant reminder to me of what she had thought and felt.

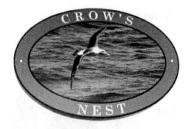

The albatross flying close to the waves, outside Beryl's room

The meaning in the images was, for Beryl, sometimes information, sometimes reminders of achievements or good times, often encouragement, perhaps consolation. There was, I think, always a sense, albeit vague, of where these works had come from, which had often been a collaborative exercise of travelling and selecting. In many of the artworks themselves, there was a sense of a pleasing and consistent whole, perhaps something of the harmony of nature. For nearly sixteen years, images largely replaced words in providing meaning for Beryl.

14

Meaning in music

All that is left for me is the music?

Fifteen years after Beryl's stroke, I wrote that music was the only thing I had left of my own life. That may sound melodramatic, but when I was part of a choral society, or an orchestra from time to time, it felt like the only time I was free to be myself. And, for a few years, I struggled even to get to rehearsals because of the full-time care and attention that Beryl needed. I did not lack for willing helpers, but coping with the practicalities was challenging. It mattered because I feel that music is what gives, and has always given, meaning to my life, and if that was to go, what would be left?

I remember that in the Author's Note at the end of his novel *An Equal Music,* Vikram Seth wrote that music was dearer to him than speech.[59] Some critics mocked him for aerated preciousness; other critics went so far as to suggest that he was simple-minded about music.[60] However, with many thousands of others, I found sufficient of interest to finish the book with some satisfaction, even if with a few reservations. And, not long ago, I found myself singing, in a chamber choir, the words of John Donne that Seth used for his title, " .. no noise nor silence, but one equal music."[61]

It would be pretentious of me to go further and to say that music means everything to me, and probably not quite true. But I am reflecting on how music touches my heart and my mind, and equally how music was important for Beryl with her progressing physical and mental problems. I have referred to music in many places in this book, apart from this chapter. It seems perhaps a little incongruous that my references to music are often, in fact, to the words that accompany, or are highlighted by, the music.

Music and rehabilitation

In the rehabilitation unit in the first few weeks after Beryl's stroke, she asked a friend to write out the words of one of her favourite hymns. Another of our musical friends sent to Beryl, in the rehabilitation unit, CDs of the music of Bach played on the piano.[62] Although Beryl had often heard me play similar recordings, I was not sure how she would respond after the stroke. In fact she played the discs regularly when she could do so herself, and later I sometimes played them for her, along with other instrumental or choral music. She herself chose music for the English church from the middle ages to the twentieth century to send to a friend for a special birthday a year or two ago.

Soon after the stroke, some friends invited us to join a meditation group. Beryl was enthusiastic, and we were both introduced through the group to music for meditation. We knew of the music from the Taizé community in France, but Margaret Rizza's music was new to us both.[63] We collected numerous recordings of her quiet songs, often based on Psalms, and versions without words for piano, guitar or chamber orchestra. Beryl used to play these repeatedly.

For several years, she was able to manage an ordinary CD player herself, but a few years ago I bought her a player produced by the Royal National Institute of Blind People, that will play automatically any disc that is inserted into the machine. Even that became too complicated for her to do, so I would put the discs on for her from time to time. As her attention span decreased, so she listened to them less frequently.

Music and memory

Much has been written about music and memory, and about music in dementia and in other mental health problems, as well as about music in people with various sorts of brain damage. So here, I am simply recording our own experiences.

Quite recently, we went to the so-called Memory Café at a local care home. The session was called *musical bingo*, and involved recognising the names of songs that were played. The names of the songs were written on cards that the teams then had to choose and place on their cardholder. I was a little dismissive in my mind, or at least not very hopeful. Beryl could not read the names. But, to my great surprise, she recognised many of the tunes. Several were old popular songs from our childhood that I thought she would never have been exposed to, certainly not since we have been married. I admit to being astonished that she knew and remembered some of those songs.

We recently attended a local concert given by talented young vocal musicians. After classical solo and ensemble pieces, the group finished with an elaborate arrangement of *Somewhere over the rainbow*. We may have watched the film *The Wizard of Oz* at home once, when the children were small, but I doubt that the song had been heard in our house for thirty years, and it was not the sort of music that Beryl's family promoted while she was growing up. But I noticed that she began to mouth the words while the group were singing. She even began to sing along – not loudly, saving my involuntary if unnecessary embarrassment – when it came to "dreams .. really do come true". An acquaintance sitting behind us noticed also. She said afterwards that she had very nearly wept to see Beryl so moved and involved, and that it had made her day.

Music visible

Over the years, Beryl and I were able to enjoy a large amount, and a great variety, of live music. She enjoyed coming to concerts in which I was singing or playing, although she needed to have someone with her.

At home, it became apparent in the last year or so that she found it very difficult to concentrate on music from CDs or on the radio. As her speech and language therapist pointed out very soon after the stroke, Beryl was a very visual person. It was good for her to have her music visible. A TV programme that she watched regularly was *Songs of Praise*. It was moving to hear, occasionally, her faint, quavering voice singing along. For recorded music, DVDs replaced CDs and most live concerts. In many ways, they were a very good substitute, because we could watch the same programme repeatedly.

Choral music in video was more attractive to Beryl than instrumental music. Our favourites were two series presented by the incomparable Simon Russell Beale. Some days, but not others, she would sit quietly and watch an hour of music from the sixteenth century.[64] Very recently, she could cope with less than the full hour, and she needed me to sit with her, but this was a treat for me rather than boring. The same musicians have produced a related video of Spanish music that is spiritual and stirring, and quite sublime, from the time of the renaissance, with its glories and terrors.[65]

Beryl was always fond of ballet. I am conscious that over the years I took her to many concerts and quite a few operas, but to very few ballets, partly because ballet has been relatively less available. But recently, we managed to get a to few live ballet productions locally, and we had several superb video recordings. When Beryl complained once about too much talking after several long phone calls, we sat and watched ballet on the television: Cinderella, with music by Prokofiev, in a beautiful and elaborate production and, of course, with no words at all. We both recovered our good spirits and watched it several times later.

Music lifts the heart

In the car, recently, we heard on the radio a piece for unaccompanied voices by Bartok. Beryl said it sounded *mournful*. It was a fair observation – some of her good words have been prompted by music. But I did not think that the music was depressing. Can mournfulness or sadness be uplifting? When I remember our experiences of the passion music of Bach and others, and of the various Requiems that I have sung recently, the answer is *Yes*.

I grew up in the post-war period in a suburban house where the piano was the feature of the lounge. We had no recorded music in the house until I was almost a teenager, but the arrival of the radiogram introduced me to music other than the piano or church organ and choir. As an accomplished teenaged pianist, my sister introduced me to a wide piano repertoire which included Mendelssohn's *Songs without Words,* while I was learning some Schubert *Lieder* with my voice teacher.

In terms of music lifting my heart, there are three specific things prominent in my memory. I can remember driving down Nathan Road in Kowloon, Hong Kong, in the mid-1980s, listening to the radio. I almost stopped when I heard, for the first time, the beginning of the String Octet,[66] which Felix Mendelssohn composed when he was just sixteen. At the beginning, there is a repeated rising and falling theme that is illustrated by the tracing (the graph in the picture) of the first

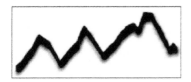 violin part. It made me think about Robert Browning's words, "a man's reach should be more than he can grasp, or what's a heaven for?"[67] When I hear this now it still encourages me to look up and forward.

Soon afterwards, I came to know Richard Strauss's *Four Last Songs.* The experts say that no one could write for the soprano voice like Strauss, and in the third of the songs,[68] which is about musing while falling asleep, there is a theme which, if traced out, has the same soaring rise and fall that I have shown in the graph above. The final appearance of the theme in the voice describes the soul wishing to soar freely, and to live deeply and a thousandfold – the final apex of the curve. I take a deep breath, and my arms and my heart lift when I hear this, no matter how often.

My third theme goes right back to the 1950s. But it stayed deep in my memory, surfacing occasionally, until forty years later when I heard it, rather incongruously, as background music in a frock shop with Beryl in Manchester. The memories came back, of my sister on the piano at home playing Chopin's second Scherzo[69] that, halfway through, has a soaring theme similar to the two I have already described. The theme is rather longer, and the shape of the curve is not quite the same, but the thrust is the same, onwards and upwards.

It is no coincidence that these three themes have a similar pattern, but I did not consciously choose them for that reason. It was only when I put them side by side from my memory that the similarities became obvious.

For me, the prime focus has always been singing, and Beryl continued over many years to come faithfully, and with great enjoyment, to my choral concerts. The physical aspects of singing are therapeutic for me. Without fail, I feel less weary these days at the end of a rehearsal than I was at the beginning. Both with singing and in the orchestra of which I was a member until recently, the collaborative group nature of the activity is an added dimension to the therapy.

Our choir director told me that the Tudor composer William Byrd wanted "to persuade every one to learn to sing."[70] His reasons included that "the exercise of singing is delightful to nature, and good to preserve the health of man". He concluded, "Since singing is so good a thing, I wish all men would learn to sing." In his liturgical environment, only men were acceptable as singers.

A rather more contemporary take on this might be from Johnny Cash's song *Daddy Sang Bass*,[71] where the chorus contains the line "Singing seems to help a troubled soul". That would be my experience too.

When I say that perhaps music is all that I have left, I am aware that this is not a small thing. Music lifts the heart: there is aspiration, and also both elation and consolation. In addition, performing music, for me and for many people, can involve travelling physically to interesting places, as well as moving the heart.

Music lifts the words

When we first came to London in the 1960s, I borrowed records and books about music from the local suburban library to maintain my peace of mind while I studied surgical anatomy and physiology full-time for six months, and Beryl worked to support us. I clearly remember coming across Leonard Bernstein's book *The Joy of Music*, based on a television series. I was struck by the powerful simplicity of Bernstein, even on the written page, walking to the front of the stage and singing operatically, rather than saying, "I love you!"

Not long after that, I came across Elgar's Sea Pictures; they still tug at my heartstrings. He set five poems with authors including Elizabeth Barrett Browning and also Adam Lindsay Gordon. At the risk of seeming maudlin, I dwell on the second, with words written by Alice Elgar, the composer's wife, with his title *In Haven (Capri)* and his verse order.[72] The first two verses are:

> Closely let me hold thy hand,
> Storms are sweeping sea and land;
> Love alone will stand.
>
> Closely cling, for waves beat fast,
> Foam-flakes cloud the hurrying blast;
> Love alone will last.

I have known and loved these songs for forty years, and as the years pass, *In Haven* seems more and more apposite to where I am now, and where we arrived at, the words unforgettable because of the music.

The poem by Herman Hesse, to which I referred earlier as a Strauss song, begins, "Now that the day has wearied me" and ends, "My unfettered soul wishes to soar up freely." The German verse is beautiful, but for me it is Strauss's music, and the violin and the voice, that lift the words literally out of this world.

Music and meaning

Keen observation over many years has led biologists to the conclusion that many animal calls are 'sung'. Anthony Storr refers to work with Gelada monkeys in Ethiopia.[73] More recent studies of white-handed gibbons[74] refer to complex songs used for communication, rather than simple calls of, for example, alarm. Esther Clarke, an anthropologist at Durham University, considers it likely that the animal noises sound similar to how humans may have communicated by song, 1.8 million years ago.

The suggestion is that human language arose out of sung communication between early humans. Margaret Rizza, the composer of meditative music, said that music is a "very strong language".[75] Everyone would agree about the strength of communication possible by music. But others go much further.

The pianist Vladimir Ashkenazy[76] said, in a filmed interview more than forty years ago, "To my mind, music is the highest expression of the human mind ... There are many things you cannot say in words because words simply don't cover everything in life."

For me, Ashkenazy's final phrase carries the day – words don't cover everything in life. I acknowledge that for me, some of the power and meaning of music comes through the specific words that I sing or hear. But listening to, or playing with, a group of instrumentalists, with no specific words at all, moves me, body and soul. And I think I have adequate evidence to say that was true for Beryl, even with her failing words and memories.

Music and acceptance – maybe rueful

A special friend introduced me to Alfred Deller singing Henry Purcell more than fifty years ago. One of the songs began with Dryden's words, "Music for a while shall all your cares beguile." Robert Schumann, before he voluntarily admitted himself to a mental asylum, wrote, "A glance at Schubert's Trio and all miserable human commotion vanishes, and the world shines in new splendour."[77] The meaning in music here is that it makes life worthwhile, or at least bearable.

Howard Goodall comments along similar lines in his excellent television series on *The Story of Music,* and the associated book. In Handel's opera *Solomon,* the Queen of Sheba sings, as she returns home, "Will the sun forget to streak eastern skies with amber ray … Then demand if Sheba's queen e'er can banish from her thought all the splendour she has seen." Goodall remarks that this is no hysterical outburst of operatic tragedy, nor is it a plaint of sentimental, self-indulgent misery. It is the mature voice of rueful acceptance. And it is the music, with the words, that make it believable and real.

Rueful acceptance – perhaps that is my situation now. We accept where we are, with some regret and ruefulness. But 'some' is an understatement; the regret and ruefulness are enormous, even overwhelming, or they would be overwhelming if I were to permit myself the space. For Beryl herself, the question became no longer rhetorical. Will the sun forget? Maybe not, but Beryl would forget. Yes she would, yes she did.

Harmony in music – and everywhere?

I am inclined, based on my own experiences and reflection, to pronounce that the meaning of life in general can be summed up in terms of music. But, irrespective of whether that sounds pretentious, I am very aware of good friends and family members, as well large proportions of all communities, for whom this is just not true. Some of my close acquaintances are passionately involved with the natural world, and not with music, and there is a limitless variety of interests among others whom I know, quite apart from the rest of humankind – including work or family or sport or hobbies.

So I wonder if a more comprehensive word like "harmony" might include all these activities and dimensions, while including music, even giving music a special place. Some might suggest "beauty", but my recent experience is that books that set out to discuss beauty tend to spend half or more of their words trying to define just what they mean by the word. To avoid a long discussion about "harmony", I propose that the word should have as broad a meaning as anyone might wish. As Howard Goodall commented, at the beginning of his television programme about harmony,[78] the word has been borrowed by everyday language to mean closeness, friendliness, human warmth, cooperation, and wellbeing.

Harmony does not necessarily involve the grand or the profound, whether in musical terms or other. Further, harmony is not necessarily on a large scale, or even particularly exciting. I thought I would show my young musician granddaughters the full orchestral score of a lively piece by Mozart that they might be able to join in, and which was one of his personal favourites.[79] I happen to be a viola player of modest accomplishment, and even I was rather surprised to see the viola part at the beginning of the piece. In the first thirty-two bars, all that the violas play is the same note 106 times. That can be harmony for you, from a viola perspective. My granddaughters were impressed, I am not sure in which way.

My focus here on harmony is much more in terms of cooperation or collaboration, fitting together and working together, than on the effect or the output. The word *ensemble* conjures up the activity well. A large proportion of singing and playing is in groups from two up to hundreds. In addition to keyboard instruments, many individual instruments played by soloists often have their own two-note or many-note harmonies.

But sometimes on instruments, including the voice, that naturally produce one note at a time, harmonies within music are implied rather than actual. This may be through sounding notes in rapid succession, or it may be much more subtle. But it does seem to me that much of what we, as human individuals and groups, are about, and perhaps what the living or even the inanimate cosmos is also about, is as much *implied harmonies* as actual harmonies. It strikes me that in the situation of Beryl and myself, our frequent disharmony still spoke of, reminded us of, hinted at, the reality and importance of harmony.

Aspiration, the ability to aspire to something broader or higher, seems to me to be part of life, and of the meaning of life. This aspiration involves creativity, innovation, the producing of harmony and the creation of new harmonies. While this may be an individual activity, I suggest that its real value comes from being shared in some way, practical or theoretical and intellectual – in cooperation, and in *ensemble*.

Silence more lovely than music?

I have recently had the pleasure of singing Bob Chilcott's setting of *The Shepherd's Carol* with a chamber choir. In Clive Sansom's words, the shepherds describe how on the hills, before they heard a voice from the sky, there was, in the calm and the stillness, "silence more lovely than music".[80] In the exquisite musical setting, the words are striking despite the fact that, like Harris's setting of Donne's words "one equal music" which I referred to above, they are not dwelt on, but passed over quite quickly. But I find myself adding a question mark: *silence more lovely than music?* Leave to poetic licence the fact that these were shepherds who were articulating beautiful words and thoughts. What sort of loveliness might silence produce or reflect? What might be the qualities, the meaning of silence?

And there is some paradox in the fact that we use – we have to use, or have the inescapable habit of using – words to describe and discuss both music and silence (and also loveliness). Furthermore, those who come to know the words "silence more lovely than music" in the twenty-first century will almost all have done so because they have heard them set to music.

I have tried to illustrate how much meaning and purpose I have found in music over very many years, and how that was also true for Beryl. But now, what meaning might there be in silence, for Beryl, for me, for all of us?

15

Meaning in silence

The inexpressible

In *Music at Night,* Aldous Huxley wrote that the things of most profound significance to the human spirit can only be experienced, not expressed. But he said that music might express the inexpressible, linking the idea to the last words of Hamlet, "The rest is silence".[81] In Hamlet's frame of mind, we might think that he was referring not just to the remainder, what was to come, but also to the ultimate of what is to come, the rest and the silence of death.

But in Beryl's situation, and our situation together, we had to deal with enforced silence, the cutting off of words, or at least of words as she would want them to be.

In our experience, there have been different types of silence. Dictionary definitions include the absence of *noise* or *sound,* but they also include the absence of *language,* which raises the question as to whether books or reading in general are silent or not. Sara Maitland points out that until relatively recently, books were usually read out loud,[82] and this chimes in with our recent experience. A leader at a Quaker camp in the United States tells how he asked the children, "Sometimes we ask you to be quiet and sometimes we ask for silence. What is the difference between quiet and silence?" A child replied, "Quiet is empty, and silence is full."[83] This aligns with "Quakerspeak", and is an example of culturally related semantics. Nevertheless, it clearly makes the point that children, as well as adults, can distinguish between varieties of silence, whatever the particular terminology might be.

Beryl was very accustomed in the past to purposeful silence. We had some experience together of meditation groups and silent retreats in Hong Kong in the 1980s. Then, in Manchester in the 1990s, when she was active in practical and academic feminist theology, she valued her silences at home. Indeed, on more than one occasion she asked, "Haven't you gone yet?", when I was a little later than usual in setting off for the medical school and leaving her in the quiet house.

The silence of watching

Beryl was always a watcher of people, and this continued after the stroke. From our house, for years she watched the cruise ships in dock and then setting off in the evenings, either shining in the summer sun, or brilliantly lit in the winter darkness – always seeming to be moving slowly and quietly.

Most of the meaning in images that I wrote of earlier arose from looking and watching, almost always in silence. Visual art, by the nature of the case, is essentially silent, except perhaps for some instances of installation art. Mark Rothko said that when he was young, in the 1920s, art was a lonely thing, by implication solitary and quiet. He added that by the end of the 1960s many artists were desperately searching for those *pockets of silence where they could root and grow*.[84]

The silence of waiting

The first meditation group that we joined was held weekly in the Convent of Poor Clares in Crossbush, near Arundel in West Sussex. Beryl talked about meditation, and about that group, in her recorded interview in 2005.

> I tried to meditate, it's the best way to do because I didn't want, I feel I can't cope with church in any reasoned thinking because all the words are going blah blah blah, they're talking non-stop, you know …
>
> And then we went and had some friends, who knocked on the door … or rang up and said, 'There's a meditation place … and then it was a wonderful time. It was a place of Clare women …

Over that time it was, oh, a year or two ... but we got into so many people who were interesting to talk with or different people in different ways and I found that a very stimulating time that was probably very good for me.

We continued going to a meditation group together until about two years ago, when the group was suspended because of health problems affecting others as well as Beryl. Beryl enjoyed the silence; she used it in her own way, as did all the other group members. By the nature of the case, even with an agreed policy (for example, using a simple word or mantra), no member of such a group knows precisely what any other member is doing in the silence.

Shortly after Beryl's stroke, I joined a Quaker meeting near where we lived. We had both had contact with Quaker meetings twenty-five years before, and I found myself very much at home in the silence. Initially, Beryl attended only occasionally, preferring to have her own time of quiet at home. But, over the past few years, she came with me, and similarly felt at home in the silence.

With both the meditation group and the Quaker meeting, there was a real sense of purpose for both of us. So there was 'meaning', in the sense of 'purpose', but for both of us there was, at least some of the time, a sense of waiting – waiting for meaning, waiting for encouragement. In the meditation group, with the aim of stilling of thoughts, it was, as it were, a long-term sort of waiting. In the Quaker group, it was a different sort of waiting, in the Quaker tradition waiting for light; the 'inward light', as the old Quakers called it. It was very much a listening silence.

The Welsh poet RS Thomas was a favourite of Beryl, who introduced me to him. His poem *Kneeling* begins with the words *Moments of great calm*. The poem talks about waiting for the message, but no particular message is referred to. Rather, the poem ends with the words *The meaning is in the waiting*.[85] Listening with Beryl a few years ago to Jim Cotter read this poem on a DVD, I noted down a thought about Job in the book in the Hebrew scriptures. Job used up all his words, and settled for silence. Silence, and silent waiting, sometimes come from running out of words as much as from deliberately putting words aside.

Thomas's poem can be read as being peaceful, but it relates to a stone church in remote northwest Wales. Even in the summer it would not have been particularly comfortable to wait there for any length of time. Waiting in silence can be peaceful or contented, but it often is focused, and it can be inescapably anxious. In my situation of caring for Beryl, when I stopped to be quiet I was, at least initially, very aware of being unquiet. It is true that Beryl had long experiences of deliberate silence, both before and after her stroke and the onset of the dementia. But recently, although she was often quiet, she was not still in her mind or body. It often seemed to me that, holding and shaking her head, and crying out, she was in fact searching for some meaning, and for some stillness that was not there.

Silence and stillness, alone or together

Being silent by oneself is clearly a very different experience from being silent as part of a group, even if what apparently, or allegedly, goes on inside the individual heart and mind is similar in both sets of circumstances.

Over recent years, Beryl began to talk about feeling lonely. She used to enjoy being by herself, but this changed as her health deteriorated. The silent groups for meditation or Quaker meetings customarily sit in circles, so each person is, in the silence, very aware of being part of a group. I am told that Zen meditation groups sometimes, or always, face outwards, but they remain group activities.

Quakers talk about 'gathered' meetings, and the concept is difficult to put into words. There is sometimes a powerful feeling of togetherness shared, as confirmed in conversation afterwards, by many or all members of the meeting. This sense of what some people would describe as 'fellowship' is perhaps unique in the Quaker context, or in group meditation, in that it arises fundamentally from the silence rather than from words or music.

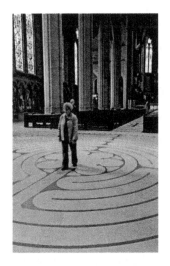

The photograph shows Beryl walking the labyrinth in Grace Cathedral in San Francisco in 2010. It was midday, so the light was coming through all the windows. The cathedral seemed almost empty, and Beryl walked alone. Quietness was all around, and stillness, despite the gentle movement. On a visit a few years earlier, other people joined Beryl and walked the labyrinth around her; there was a clear overall sense of purposeful and shared silence. There was almost palpable meaning in the silence for Beryl.

There are other examples of what might be called 'populated silence'. One, which is experienced in certain classical or formal music events, is noted by Vikram Seth[86]: the strange silence of a large audience gathered in a concert hall, waiting for or immediately after a performance. Just before Beryl's stroke, she came with me to a performance of Schubert's song cycle *Die schöne Müllerin* in London. The last of the twenty songs describes quietly and sadly the death in the stream of the rejected lover. On this particular occasion, after the final notes died away on the piano, there was more than a minute's complete stillness: the two performers and the two hundred listeners together in silence; a remarkable tribute to the composer and to the performers, and also to the involvement of the audience. Traditional minutes of silence for remembrance of war or death or tragedy similarly illustrate the power, the 'meaning' of shared silence.

Perhaps a little paradoxically, in both the meditation group as referred to in Beryl's interview above, and in the Quaker meetings, there has always been a lot of talk, especially after the meetings. This can be part of the enjoyment of the group, although it is not the group's primary activity. So silence goes together with, and derives at least some of its 'meaning' from, surrounding noise or language or words or music. Part of the meaning of engaging with the natural world, which I referred to earlier in discussing images, often relates to stillness and calm. In fact, nature is not usually completely silent, but the outdoors is also not normally noisy and loud, and the walker or climber is often at some remove from the sounds of life. I am reminded of my walk through the wheatfield that I described in the first chapter of this book.

What sort of meaning in silence?

In contrast to music, meaning in silence has probably been more important for Beryl than for me, for many years. If I sat with her and held her left hand – she did not really register feeling in the right hand – and said nothing, did that have meaning? I think so. When we walked together, I held her by her left hand; it meant we were together, with me supporting or guiding. If I just sat alongside her, that meant companionship, I hope, provided that I could avoid using my smartphone too much.

When Huxley wrote that silence and music express the inexpressible, I think that he had in mind rather grander concepts than sitting companionably, or a short walk. But if the silence is enforced, and the damaged brain cannot formulate, let alone express, abstract or elaborate ideas, I think it may be not demeaning but rather life-affirming to settle for very simple and basic, but still inexpressible, experiences. In the silences of watching, and of waiting, there have in the past been broader and deeper experiences. They have, I think, shaped Beryl and me, even though she may not have been able to recollect them.

So is meaning there, even if it is not articulated? I think the answer, from my reflections about images and music and silence, is clearly *Yes*. I can see that there is 'respite' for me in the music and in the silence, and in sleep. But I am aware that I am expressing my own view. Beryl became unable to understand the question, even less so to formulate an answer. But meaning for me, and meaning for her, have been intertwined, and this connection is not unique to us, and not unique to our joint predicament of failing mental and physical health.

I think that all the questions and answers about meaning are gathered up in the whole encompassing business of caring, in the broadest sense.

16

The meaning is in the caring

Caring in context

In the stories that I have told thus far, I have aimed, first, to spell out in detail the nature of the disabilities caused by stroke, dysphasia and dementia. I have also intended to acknowledge how well Beryl coped, and to record how I tried to cope. Secondly, I have aimed to set out both the context and the challenge of looking for meaning, including showing why I felt, and still feel, the need for meaning or purpose or value.

In writing this chapter, I began with my feelings and my intuition that the whole business of caring, in a specific health context but also in its broadest sense, must be intimately involved with the purpose and meaning of our lives, and much more generally with the meaning of life as a whole. In trying to justify my wide and general proposition, I will add to our own experiences my reflection on the thoughts and experiences of many other people down the ages, including some who have had similar experiences to ours.

Beryl as a carer – what she cared about

I am aware that while this book has not been negative about Beryl, the force and effect of her illnesses and disabilities have dominated much of what I have written about her.

But it was not always like that, and a good demonstration is to report on some of the tributes paid to her at the memorial service held after her death.

> Beryl was, above all things, an encourager; she was so generous in heaping praise on her friends. What a gift she had, to say without the slightest tinge of a grudge, or envy, that someone was brilliant at doing something, or looked especially nice; she was observant of all the little things, and was quick to make her pleasure in others known.

> Beryl was a remarkable woman whose support for men, women, boys and girls was completely and utterly abundant.

> She was an organised and determined woman whose, steely determination was fuelled by her own personal pain, the injustices she had experienced, and those she had witnessed.

We always admired and appreciated her wise counsel, ready sense of humour, indomitable spirit and desire to communicate with all her friends.

She was vivacious and welcoming; she never wavered in her welcome.

Beryl cared deeply for her friends and family, and for wider issues. Hospitality was part of that care, especially, she said, if someone else was doing the cooking. Her smile, on which everyone commented, was a manifestation of her interest in, and care for, all those around her.

Our grandchildren said,

Whenever we visited her, her whole face lit up with happiness. When we were around, she was always laughing and smiling. Gran was always a lovely kind person.

Our own adult children said:

Mum was gentle, warm and kind; she was hardworking, determined and organized; she was caring, loving and compassionate; she was supportive, generous and thoughtful.

She was brave through the years since her stroke, and she continued to care for others; she even comforted us when we were distressed by her disabilities.

We could see her sociable nature endure right to the end: with a smile she thanked the young student paramedic who helped take her to the hospital for the last time; she thanked the health care assistant in the emergency department; with a smile, she thanked the porters and nursing staff who took her to the ward.

Beryl's history as a carer went back more than fifty years before her stroke. Following her father losing most of his sight in an accident, when she was only seven years old and her sister was only two, Beryl became, in many ways, a child carer. She was a dutiful, diligent and capable child, and took a good share of the caring over the years.

As she grew older, she helped her father with the plans of the houses he continued to build, and in dealing with his subcontractors and his accounts. She had become a university student before she obtained her driving licence on her seventeenth birthday, and she immediately became the family chauffeur both for business and for pleasure.

Of course, her mother and sister, between them, carried the majority of the burden as the years went by, but Beryl continued to feel the effects of the weight of responsibility all her life.

In addition to family and school teaching, Beryl took on caring and support roles in Hong Kong – including involvement in a women's refuge – and in Manchester. I feel the need to acknowledge and affirm this, at the risk of appearing to minimise it by being very brief, especially about our family. But Beryl can speak at least a little for herself, in terms of things that she wrote, or that I can remember her saying.

Beryl said to me not long ago that she would like to go to see her sister in Australia, and to help with her sister's husband, who was in a care home with dementia. She did not remember how she scarcely coped with the last long-haul flights we took more than three years previously.

Beryl's awareness of loss was sometimes coupled with memories of being a helpful and caring person. "All my life was helping and helping," she said, adding, "and now nobody cares". Another time she said, "I try and I try and I try." But often she mentioned the loss of her roles and abilities in so many words. "I used to be OK but now I've lost all the ideas ... I can't do things properly anymore." She even said one day, echoing what used to be called the 'general confession', "I have not done the things that I used to have done." She once said, "I've lost my faculties." Another time simply, "I can't fathom ..." And another time, poignantly (an overworked word but unavoidable), "It's just that I can't understand my mind."

In late 2014, as we enjoyed finding our way around Venice, Beryl said to a travelling companion, "Stuart knows everything. He is loving and caring and generous, and I love him." After a month in the care home, she said to one of the staff as I came in, "That's my number one." But such affirmation as there is for me in instances like these makes me feel tearful rather than gratified.

So we have had occasional moments of remembered affection and enjoyment. And I remind myself that Beryl has been a willing, able and caring partner for me for very many years. I remember those words that Thomas Cranmer apparently conjured out of his fertile imagination and his own experience, including marriage: "the mutual society, help, and comfort that the one ought to have of the other, both in prosperity and adversity."[87]

In the years before the stroke, Beryl spoke and wrote many times about the contributions of women especially, but not only, in the church. On one memorable occasion, she drew attention to how the contribution of women is often compared and contrasted with, even turned into a competition with, the contribution of men. She passionately made the case for what she called "side by sideness". This was a plea for women and men to think and work side-by-side. Her ideas came partly from consideration of the roles of women in society and in the church, but she wished to see the ideas applied at all levels including, but not restricted to, personal relationships and the family. Beryl's principle of side by sideness was not so much about couples as about collaboration and community.

For Beryl, it seems a reasonable summary to say that the meaning of her life was in the caring, often needing to be backed up by hard thinking and good organisation.

Evolution and costly cooperation

I hear, from time to time, a question about whether Beryl's illnesses, or other people's, are part of some grand plan. My response is always a firm *No*, certainly in relation to any way in which the word "plan" is normally used. But I do see them as part of a comprehensive system that is usually called evolution. Natural selection has shaped the development of our human bodies, and I wrote something about this in relation to heart rhythms and the functions of the brain in the early chapters of this book.

Human society, as well as human language, anatomy and physiology, has been formed and shaped through natural selection. The evolution of parental care, mostly maternal, seems not difficult to understand, and I would say that hunter-gatherers, both males and females, were providers, and can thus be broadly considered as carers.

A year or two before her stroke, I introduced Beryl to the book *An Intelligent Person's Guide to Ethics* by Mary Warnock, and she was very interested. Warnock proposes that ethical thinking arises when people begin to see that their own society, and then human beings at large, are all in the same boat; it is a precarious boat that will sink if there is no cooperation among those who are on board.[88] Warnock argues that this opens up the possibility of 'altruism', an idea that she elaborates in a later book. She considers that an essential feature of morality is the ability to treat others as having a greater need than oneself. The morally good person, she says, must be prepared, at least sometimes, to postpone his or her own interests in order to protect or promote the interests of other people.[89]

In the philosophical, sociological and biological literature, there is much discussion and disagreement about 'altruism'. That discussion includes the literature relating to the evolutionary development of altruism, which is sometimes called "evolutionary cooperation". Confusingly, what "cooperation" means, in that context, is what I prefer to call "costly cooperation". The evolution of cooperation, in the usual sense of mutuality, is said to be not difficult to explain. But Coakley defines the more complex and costly idea in terms of evolutionary fitness, with one entity gaining fitness while another entity suffers loss of fitness.[90] The argument from mathematical biology is that evolutionary benefit can follow from cooperative acts with various levels of reciprocity. Nowak says that evolution is remarkably constructive because it can generate cooperation in a competitive world.[91] It is interesting, and important, to see that this principle of cooperation is said to apply to evolving populations of organisms of all complexities. The reader can then see some point in restricting the word 'altruism' to conscious, motivated cooperation, in human groups and possibly others.

Without wishing to make too great a claim about the use of words, I think it is reasonable to say that the idea of costly cooperation, or altruism, in human society could be called, if not simply 'helping', then perhaps 'caring'. This may be a roundabout way to add further support to my assertion that the meaning of life is in the caring; it seems to me to be of fundamental importance.

In the context of caring, it is interesting and important how words are used. I can remember being surprised that the expression "looked after children" became an official description in the UK Children Act in 1989. But I could see that even though the expression seemed rather informal, it was useful and practical, and non-judgemental. And it emphasised how many young people needed to be "in care" in one way or another.

In discussions with some professionals about dementia care, I have been impressed with their concern about the quality of client care, but also about the quality of the care which the staff receive from their managers. In particular, I was struck by how one professional expressed the view that 'caring' is more *sacrificial* than 'altruism'. It is true that many aspects of 'altruism' in academic discussions do not involve close relationships. But I was impressed by this professional person saying, based on many observations of mother-daughter and husband-wife situations, that "People who care from the heart have a much more difficult time." It was this professional who wanted to feel free to talk with carers like me about values such as 'love', and also about 'sacrifice'. Compassion, sympathy and empathy are all words and ideas potentially involved in these discussions. Discussions of subtle differences of meaning are interesting, but an unaffordable luxury for those actually involved in the caring. I am content to say that the sort of caring that I am talking about here takes place within a relationship of some sort, and that the caring is costly. In the case of Beryl and myself, there has been a long-standing and mutual relationship, and that applies to a very large number of people in similar situations to ours.

Global ethics

I could try to put this into a global context by quoting statistics from a variety of countries. I have referred earlier to groups such as Stroke Associations, and Alzheimer's or Dementia Associations, which exist in many countries, and from whose websites or publications these statistics can be obtained. Instead,

I want to briefly discuss global attitudes to what I am simply calling 'caring'.

The book *A Global Ethic*[92] has, as the third of its six declarations, "a principle which is found and has persisted in many religious and ethical traditions of humankind for thousands of years: What you do not wish done to yourself, do not do to others. Or, in positive terms: What you wish done to yourself, do to others! This should be the irrevocable, unconditional norm for all areas of life, for families and communities, for races, nations, and religions."[93]

This specific global ethics publication came from the so-called "Parliament of the World's Religions", an extremely broad international group. A non-religious code of global ethics has also been put forward.[94] The ten humanist principles are: dignity, respect, tolerance, sharing, no domination, no superstition, conservation, no war, democracy, and education.

There is a very large overlap between these 'religious' and 'humanist' views. The sixth humanist principle asks people to rely on reason, logic and science to understand the universe and to solve life's problems. But I think that most of the 'religious' groups would not have many problems with that, provided that imagination and the philosophical aspects of science were permitted in the mix with proper reflection and accountability. It is widely acknowledged that for both religious and political ideologies, there has been some inconsistency about whether the 'golden rule' should be applied only to 'people like us'.

I think that both these views of global ethics include what I am calling 'caring', and extend the idea very broadly to include all the natural world.

Care ethics

Some years before her stroke, I introduced Beryl to several texts in bioethics. There was considerable interest not only in what "life" meant, but also in what "value" meant. I learnt much from *The Value of Life*[95] and its author, as I studied and worked with him. But, from the outset, I had some questions about how important a place language seemed to be given as the basis of people valuing themselves. Those ideas continued to be important as Beryl's health problems progressed.

There was mutuality for us in that in the few years before her stroke, Beryl introduced me to relatively new aspects of ethics during her Master's degree programme in theology with feminist studies.

Beginning in 1982, Carol Gilligan wrote about "a different voice". She pointed out that in ethical theories, men's experience and thought was taken to stand for all human experience and thought. She wrote that what emerged repeatedly in interviews with women was a responsibility to care – to discern and alleviate the real troubles in the world.[96] She added that the ideal of care was an activity of relationship, of seeing and responding to need.

This is a world-view, not just a consideration of isolated couples or groups. She wrote about the ethics of justice and care, the ideals of human relationships. "Care ethics" was the name given later to this perspective; the emphasis was on broadening and combining perspectives and especially on mutuality. Fundamentally, Gilligan thought, the most basic questions about how to live were questions about human relations.

Another book to which Beryl introduced me was a reader in feminist ethics, particularly a chapter by Christine Gudorf. This chapter rose largely from her challenging parenting experiences, including adopting two young children who, in her own words, were medically handicapped. In this context of demanding care, Gudorf chose to write not only about *love* but also about *sacrifice*. She made the case that all love involves sacrifice, and that all love is also directed at mutuality.[97]

Further thoughts in this direction have come to me through Raimond Gaita's writings, specifically his book *"A Common Humanity – thinking about love and truth and justice"*, based on his own experiences, and those of his family and community, including the Holocaust. He points out how the language traditionally used in ethics and morality has failed to cover all of life as it is actually lived. To the idea of *love*, he adds that of *mystery*. But he is critical in thinking that most philosophies do not seem to see the need for mystery.[98]

So I think that 'ethics' and 'caring' are closely aligned. I am not meaning to confine my remarks about caring, and about ethics, to couples, although of course many of my own thoughts and experiences arise in that way. As I have said, everyone cares, in one way or another, for family or friends or acquaintances, even strangers. In any of these situations, whole-hearted caring raises questions and provides some answers about meaning. But caring, especially perhaps extreme caring, also introduces aspects of what Gaita called mystery. Andrew Miller wrote of one of his characters that her affliction flushed out triviality and made her acquaintances into mystics and philosophers.[99]

Achievative or affiliative?

When Beryl was able to study for a diploma in personnel management, thirty-five years ago, she discussed many modules with me, and introduced me to some new jargon. Working people, perhaps people in general, could be divided (her tutors said) into two categories: those who were achievative and those who were affiliative. The first was a new word for me, and it does not seem to be in standard or common use now, but the contrast being made was fairly obvious.

Such contrasts can be seen among work colleagues and acquaintances, and family. But I have tried to make clear that I draw no comparisons of virtue or morals between those who are natural-born carers, and those who are not. Even if we accept this achievative-affiliative distinction, the wellbeing of our society requires that there should be much achievement in terms of creativity and originality in science and in the humanities – and in health and social care.

In any case, in the "caring professions", as in other workplaces, some people are more empathetic than others. Achievements and feelings may be separable, but in actual caring, feelings and words need to be supported by actions, and are nothing without actions. Down the ages, many agencies, including political, military, educational, and religious (including the family of TS Eliot, in whose poetry Beryl was intensely interested), have had mottoes or guides summed up as "actions not words".

So, by 'caring' (probably by 'loving' also) I mean primarily 'doing' rather than 'feeling'. It is possible, of course, to do what might be 'caring' without much sympathy, because of fatigue or distraction or even because of personality. But, as we all know, caring in an unfeeling way can cause problems, especially in care homes.

Duty and joy, love and trial

I was aware quite soon after Beryl's stroke that a phrase kept running through my mind: "it is our duty and our joy". The phrase was published in 1973, having been produced by a committee revising the Book of Common Prayer. It seemed to sum up the ambivalence of my feelings about our situation. There was some sort of joy in caring for her, as well as a sense of duty – not a heavy duty, but nevertheless the phrase that came to mind seemed appropriate.

I think it is true that I have rarely dwelt on the 'joy' idea. It was not always easy to see which part of our experience fitted that word, but certainly there was, at times, a sense of pleasure and satisfaction in supporting Beryl, and succeeding in giving her some measure of pleasure. I have remembered from time to time the words of the Dalai Lama that I have quoted earlier. What makes true happiness: money, a big house, accomplishment, friends, or compassion and good heart?

A different expression of the contrasts in experiences like ours puts the words 'love' and 'trial' together. That interesting, if imperfect, guru from the 1970s and 1980s Scott Peck defined love as the will to extend one's self for the purpose of nurturing one's own or another's growth.[100] A simple version of love as "wishing the other well" may not capture the full force, but is easier to grasp than his original, which includes the word 'spiritual' used in a general sort of way. Peck emphasises that love is an action, an activity, and he emphasises that all love contains the risk of loss.

About ten years before Beryl's stroke, I was privileged to sing evensong at Great Malvern Priory as part of a visiting choir, which included my daughter. This visit was memorable for the music, but also because I found, in the graveyard, the headstone for Annie Darwin:

> Anne Elizabeth Darwin
> Born March 2, 1841
> Died April 23, 1851
> A dear and good child

Annie was the second child, and eldest daughter, of Charles Darwin. She died, probably of consumption, while in Great Malvern, having gone there to take the waters with her parents. However, her father had returned home to Kent a few days earlier. One week later, he wrote a memorial. The final paragraph begins, "We have lost the joy of the Household ... she must have known how we loved her."[101]

Ten years after Annie's death, Charles Darwin wrote to JD Hooker, a great botanist and his greatest friend, whose son had the scarlet fever. The letter ended:

> Much love much trial, but what an utter desert is life without love.
> God Bless you | C. D.[102]

I have repeated to myself, and to others, many times over the years: "much love, much trial", which seems another apposite summary of how Beryl's life and mine have worked out. But I would always continue with the rest of the perceptive words of the great man, who was very far from being a dry scientist: "what an utter desert is life without love."

Imperfect or impotent caring

I am very aware that over the past few years there have been many occasions on which I have done my best, but it has not been good enough. My point is not that my contribution was complained about, although I have said earlier that was the case from time to time. It is rather that, objectively, I could not single-handed, or sometimes even with help, provide the type, or standard, of care that Beryl needed. Also, I have talked about burnout. Every so often, I would feel not just that I could not go on, but also that I did not want to go on.

I sat by her bedside in the care home. She looked at me and said, "You're a good man." But it was only the next day, when I left after a short, tiring visit, that she sharply said, "Don't run away." My performance in caring was of variable standard, and often imperfect.

In the last few months before she was admitted to the care home, I felt it was a red-letter day when I went the whole day without raising my voice. My aim in life used to be to care for her, to entertain her, to make her laugh every day, to hold her hand when she was dying. (My family had heard me say this, and reminded me later that it did not turn out that way.) My aim reduced to this each day – not to shout at her. I was not sure whether I was comforted when some younger friends told me that their daily aim, relating to their growing children, was just the same; not to shout at them. I am told that Homer Simpson said, "You tried your best and you failed miserably. The lesson is: Never try." Black humour is one way for me to try to deal with these harshest of realities.

My on-going feeling of responsibility for Beryl was tied to the feeling that I had on the first day of the stroke; I wished her not to be 'comfortless'. My family pointed out that in the last week or two, she had perhaps become beyond comforting.

So my experience was that caring could become both inadequate and ineffective. And I now find that the situations about which I most care, apart from Beryl, and after she has passed beyond care, are situations where I can usually do nothing. This is often because it is not appropriate for me to interfere, as it were, or again where there is no feasible intervention. Friends have pointed out to me that to listen is in fact to do something rather than nothing, and this has been helpful.

My relationship with Beryl became attenuated because of illness and time, and my caring became increasingly imperfect or impotent. I am very aware that relationships change over time for many people – even fail – and that for them, too, the whole business of 'caring', in however general a way that word may be used, may become imperfect or impotent. I know that I am one of many who cannot claim that, over the years, our caring, attention, affection and loyalty to our partner, our family, or our neighbours, have been beyond criticism. This is quite different from me doing my best and still failing; I need to acknowledge that sometimes I didn't, in fact, do my best. Imperfect caring could, I suppose, be considered the norm, and we all have to deal with that as best we can. From time to time relationships do break down in one way or another; that seems sometimes unavoidable.

I need therefore to acknowledge that situations have arisen for me, and may have arisen for others, where my assertion that the meaning is in the caring might be questioned. My response for myself, and possibly for others, is that there *was* meaning in whatever caring was achieved, and that failure or decreasing effectiveness of the caring does not deny the general principle. I would say, further, that other people and things are now what I care for, or am beginning to care for, now that my caring space and my caring opportunities are opening up again. This would, I hope, be a common experience.

Caring, loss and death

In the final stages of revising this chapter, Beryl died, rather unexpectedly. During the second admission to hospital in her four-month residence at the care home, she succumbed to a chest infection that had built up, with her decreasing mobility, over several weeks.

'Death' is the last chapter in the outstanding book by Nick Lane[103] about what he calls the ten greatest inventions of evolution. Lane points out the basic fact, that without death there would be no natural selection, no evolution.

For humankind, the problem is that there are many genes, or combinations of genes, that for various reasons are good for something in early life, especially related to reproduction, but produce illnesses later in life. Lane considers that *diseases of ageing* probably cannot be eradicated, but that the general phenomenon of the *ageing of cells* in the human body, with complex biochemical causes, might be modified. Genetic differences are well known, for example, in parts of Japan where, after age fifty, some groups have fewer than half the health problems that the rest suffer, and are twice as likely to live to a healthy 100. They do not live to very much more than 100; the biological ageing process still exists even though it is delayed.

In the context in which I am writing, the final paragraph of Lane's book is poignant. The chances are we will never live for ever, nor would we really wish to, says Lane, fairly incontrovertibly. In particular, he points out, the most specialised cells of all are the neurons of the human brain, and when they die, they are not replaced. Lane suggests that if, one day, we succeed in engineering a pool of neuronal stem cells to replace dead brain cells, we must surely replace our own experience – our own memories, perhaps even our own words – into the bargain. He thinks that our brains are, in principle, not replaceable. I frame a question for myself based on Sally Magnusson's book about her mother's dementia: where do memories go? I will make space for that question in the subsequent book.

Beryl's death, then, is part of evolved biological and human experience. I need to think this and to feel it. My sense of sadness and loss has a framework. What more meaning there might be in the death of Beryl, and the deaths of others, I will also leave to the companion book.

But, as to the everyday, loss comes and it comes in stages. On handing over all Beryl's day-to-day practical care to the care home, compared with having help with some of the care while she was still at home, I went from being a carer back to being 'just' a husband. And then came the final loss of Beryl's rather sudden death. But there was relief with the loss; relief for her, and for me and the family. When friends asked me, I responded that I felt that I was near the end of my bereavement rather than at the beginning. Much, probably most, of the loss and grieving had already taken place before Beryl died.

I am aware that my situation of loss is far from unique. I am also aware of concern amongst family and friends for me. I am now, to some extent, in the position of being cared for. On reflection, this has been true ever since I became a 'carer'. I have acknowledged that, for Beryl and myself, even as her health problems progressed, there was still some aspect of mutuality. The fact that she depended on me was an aspect of her caring about me, even if 'caring about' and 'caring for' are not quite the same.

I think that this past and present mutuality is part of what made me feel, rather than just theorise, that the meaning is in the caring. Although 'caring' became focused on me doing things *for* her, I remember often thinking that I would much rather be doing things *with* her. On any day, when I managed to do things with her – things we both enjoyed, such as going to gardens or garden centres – that was a real positive, and that continued even for the short time that she was in the care home.

In earlier years, even up to just a few months before Beryl was admitted to the care home, we managed to travel together within Europe and the United Kingdom. At least before her admission, we both enjoyed eating and drinking together, even with me helping her eat. But in the final few months, I noticed that when people came into her room – even our own children and grandchildren – Beryl would look at me, sometimes over their shoulder, with uncertainty and needing some reassurance. I really did have to do many things for her rather than with her. But when she looked at me like that, I was more conscious of the reality and persistence of the bond between us, rather than of a burden.

My conclusion here is, therefore, that despite loss and separation, there are always some broad aspects of care and mutuality that remain, even though they may need to be reconstructed or reinterpreted. My experience, our experience, has been that *mutual* caring establishes the fundamental 'meaning' of caring. Getting out of balance, as it were, with care, for example with one of the individuals in a relationship having to do all the caring, does not invalidate the principle; mutuality remains as the underlying concept.

It could, I suppose, seem harsh to imply that if there is no caring, there is no meaning. I have acknowledged that my new situation, after Beryl's recent death, has meant thinking differently about caring. But I am content to maintain that meaning is in relationships – relationships of caring. Each of us needs to rise to the challenge of finding out for ourselves what, in practice, our relationships are, and where our caring lies, and what is the meaning in it all.

17

You have to go on

How long?

We were in the transit lounge at the airport in Los Angeles, on the way back from another visit to my mother in Australia. Beryl was in a wheelchair provided by the airline, to make the transfers easier and quicker. I noticed a man also pushing his wife in a wheelchair. They had been on our plane, and he seemed rather grumpy, while she was making noises but not saying anything very coherent. So I spoke to the man in a companionable, co-traveller sort of way, if that is possible in airports.

I said that it was now three years after Beryl's stroke, and that we had enjoyed the flight. He said, confirming his apparent grumpiness by his tone of voice, "We have been like this for sixteen years." The only word that I can use to describe my feeling on hearing this is 'gobsmacked'. I can remember feeling appalled, and rather panicked, at the idea that this sort of situation could drag on and on and on. A moment of medical reflection might have produced the thought, "Of course," but mine was no rational response.

In our sixteenth year

I wrote this chapter while Beryl was in the care home, a few months before she died unexpectedly. We were in our sixteenth year of caring after the stroke. I have written, in the previous chapter, about caring and loss, and I acknowledge that you have to go on *after* your loss. But I have chosen to leave the rest of the words of this chapter unchanged, rather than update them. They reflect my feelings at the time, but I believe they also reflect the situation of very many other people in this country, and around the world, who are grappling with the effects of stroke and dementia.

I can't go on like this

Repeatedly, over the past few years, I have found myself thinking, "I don't want to do this any more" or "I can't, we can't, go on like this."

That idea occurs in Samuel Beckett's play *Waiting for Godot*.[104] In the situation of what I suppose might be called expectant confusion the idea of 'not going on like this' is not quite brushed aside, but the retort is not encouraging.

Then I hear people quoting similar words at the end of another of Beckett's rather impenetrable works, *The Unnamable*.[105] The speaker says that they can't go on, and then immediately adds that they will go on. The basic idea, which I have translated colloquially from Beckett's French original and used as my theme for this book and in its title, is that 'you have to go on'. The words become me speaking to myself.

And as Beckett's speaker says, that seems to sum everything up: you have to go on, that's all I know. These ideas, profound if obscure, have become a focus, even an obsession for me as I have reflected and written over the past fifteen years about our predicament, and the similar situations of so many people.

The feelings bound up in these words may be those of persistence or stubbornness, or of regret, even resentment at times. But I do not think that detracts from the value of what carers do, nor of course from the value of the persistence of those who are cared for. You have to go on.

Why do you have to go on?

A little before Beryl was first admitted to hospital, at the end of 2014, one of my friends asked me, "Why do you have to go on?"

She did not mean that I would give up caring; she meant that I could pass over the procedures of caring to some other agency. That idea had been, for years, at the bottom of my wish list, but I knew that Beryl's sister cared for her husband as she always had, even though he was in an institution. Thousands of carers do so, and I thought that I could probably do that too.

Eventually I did concede defeat, and Beryl became a long term resident in a care home. But you still have to go on, in one way or another.

She has to go on

What she has wanted – often sadly, sometimes despairingly – is *not* to go on. Sometimes she says, "I will be dead." More often, she wants to go *back* – to *home*, to the old days "when I was young."

Near the end of their life, some people have been able to reflect on their experiences, in writing or in speech, with great perception and clarity. Clive James wrote of feeling the paradox that his death was something he had to live with.[106] Dementia is different in that the individual sufferer cannot usually verbalise their experiences, or even be fully aware of them. Terry Pratchett is a notable exception. One of his late pieces was entitled, "I'm slipping away a bit at a time … and all I can do is watch it happen."[107] A few other people with early dementia have managed to record their experiences and thoughts. But usually, it is an observer or a carer who observes and thinks and writes.

In the meantime, and for who knows how long, Beryl either cannot clearly express her desires, or else is quite unable to put them into action. She just has to go on.

We have to go on

I need to be honest with myself, and with any reader who has persisted this far. My ideas about finding meaning – in images, in music, in silence, and especially in the caring – have needed to be tested and tried, and they have indeed been pushed to their limits.

I have explained that much of my consolation, my meaning, my pleasure, comes from music in one way or another. As I write, Beryl and I can still sit together and watch DVDs of music, and also about art; the television set is a shared interest.

In one of the very early episodes of the TV medical drama *Grey's Anatomy,* a young man with a brain tumour is warned that an operation might cause him to lose his memories. His wife says earnestly, "I'll remember for both of us." I was touched when I saw that, but I was not at all sure that it was realistic, or that it was in any way reassuring or comforting to the man who was the patient.

In the final series of the Swedish TV detective series *Wallander*, he is shown sinking slowly into the forgetfulness of Alzheimer's disease. A specially composed song in English covers the end credits of the final episode with the words, "When there's so much darkness closing in ..."[108] Similarly, the last Wallander book *The Troubled Man* describes a darkness in which there were no lamps to light.[109] At the end of the final television episode, Kurt Wallander says to his colleagues, including his daughter, "For as you already know or suspect or feel I have – sorry – Alzheimer's. You may have seen me irritable and annoyed. I forget things, important and unimportant. But I hope you will remember – because I won't – the good times we had." It seemed somehow different when the individual sufferer said that for themself.

While things stay as they are now, I can take Beryl out in the car from the care home and, with the wheelchair, do some of the simple things we used to do together. I will remember the good times we had, and she will, for the time being, remember some of those times too.

In the care home, the situation continues to be what I call extreme caring. The carers are *caring*, as am I, and as are the relatives and friends of other residents whom I observe day after day. There are even a few couples among the residents, who clearly still care for each other within the limits of their fading abilities. So my conclusion expands a little: the meaning that remains is still in the caring, and there is meaning also in the carers, and in their remembrances.

And music can have the last word, or almost. There is Bach and Byrd and Rizza that Beryl likes to listen to in her room, albeit for ever shorter periods of time. The other day, while I was giving Beryl her lunch in the care home, I realised that the radio in the background was playing the waltz from Tchaikovsky's opera Eugene Onegin. I could not help smiling. There were eight residents, including one couple lunching together, and two carers, and me. Would that some or all of us had had the heart, and the body and mind to go with it, to get up and waltz together! We settle for the ever-slowing waltz of caring.

I wrote earlier that I am comfortable with people using as broad a definition as they wish of 'caring'. I am also comfortable with people using as broad a definition of 'love' as they wish. In the second of Elgar's Sea Pictures, to which I referred earlier, the words are from a poem written by his wife Alice. The refrains are:

Love alone will stand
Love alone will last
Love alone will stay (which was also her original title of the poem)

Mary Shelley wrote that "love will render loss endurable".[110] I am not as sure about that as I am about Alice Elgar's view in her poem and the song. Jung's contribution was to write that "meaning makes a great many things endurable, perhaps everything."[111] Love will last, will endure, but I think that there is absolutely no option, no alternative – the loss also endures, goes on, whether or not it seems bearable, and the search for meaning goes on too.

We have to go on.

Rage or consolation?

I would not want my reflections on the experiences of ourselves, and many like us, to be inappropriately reassuring or consoling. I do not wish to conclude by appearing to say that I have provided a prescription or a solution for living with these sorts of problems. I cannot honestly have an up-beat ending.

Rather, when I am honest, behind the heartache and the tears, and at the same time as I go on caring for as long as I can, I know that I rage, rage against the dying of the light. Any consolation that goes with that comes from knowing that innumerable others – sufferers and carers – rage with me, and that, at the same time as I am raging, many people are caring for me as well as for her.

The final words and revisions of this book have been written after the white heat of extreme caring suddenly stopped. But the effects of these experiences, on me and on my family, fade slowly, and are revived by the reflection and writing.

At the end, I know you have to go on – but that's not really all I know.

Acknowledgements

I am grateful for support and encouragement during the past sixteen years, especially from my family, and also from many friends. I have valued professional support from staff of Age Concern Hampshire and of Hartford Care (now The Cinnamon Care Collection), and especially of St Mary's GP Surgery, Southampton and of the Admiral Nursing Service, Southampton.

In revising the material for this book, I have appreciated input from my family, and also from many friends and colleagues, especially Karen Cotton, David Deboys, Margaret Fuller, Betty Lanchester, Liz Parry, John Vickerman, Linda Watson, and Ann Williams.

Notes and Sources

Sources referred to in the numbered notes are listed below, with other comments. All websites referred to were accessible in June 2016.

These details are also available at the internet address www.donnan.eu/extreme where there are active web links to books, articles, illustrations and music. On the website, all the illustrations from this book are available in their original colour.

1. The National Stroke Strategy policy document published by the UK Department of Health in 2007 can be viewed online at http://clahrc-gm.nihr.ac.uk/wp-content/uploads/DoH-National-Stroke-Strategy-2007.pdf

2. Angela Cotter was carrying out a Quaker-related research project. The interview transcript is used with her agreement.

3. Stroke Association UK is at www.stroke.org.uk while many other countries have national and local groups supporting people with strokes and supporting stroke research.

4. One of many sources is RG Loosemore: The inversion hypothesis: a novel explanation for the contralaterality of the human brain. *Bioscience Hypotheses* Volume 2, Issue 6, 2009, Pages 375–382. Accessible online

at http://www.hy-ls.org/index.php/hyls/article/download/14/14-115-1-PB.pdf

5.   Norman Doidge. *The Brain That Changes Itself: Stories of Personal Triumph from the Frontiers of Brain Science*, Penguin Books, 2007.

6.   Maryanne Wolf. Proust and the Squid: *The Story and Science of the Reading Brain*, Icon Books, 2008.

7.   Frances Spufford. *Unapologetic: Why, despite everything, Christianity can still make surprising emotional sense*, Faber & Faber, 2012.

8.   Samuel Beckett. *Endgame*. Faber & Faber, 2009. The French original was entitled *Fin de partie;* first performed in 1957.

9.   Stuart Donnan. *Faith when words and memory fail: reflections on a spiritual life with stroke and dementia*, forthcoming.

10. Terry Eagleton. *The Meaning of Life: a very short introduction*, OUP, 2008.

11. Visit of the Dalai Lama as reported in the Independent newspaper (London) on 4 March 2014.

12. Alasdair MacIntyre. *After Virtue: a study in moral theory*, Duckworth, 2nd ed. 1985, page 218; also Raymond Gaita. *Good and Evil*, Macmillan, 1991, pages 134-5.

13. Jennie Erdal. *What's the Big Idea?* Financial Times 7 April 2012, at https://next.ft.com/content/1cc50e4c-7d81-11e1-81a5-00144feab49a

14. From the UK: Myint and colleagues. *Postgrad Med J.* Sep 2006; 82(971): 568–572 (summary at http://pmj.bmj.com/content/82/971/568.abstract). From Italy: Beghi. *Neurology* April 8, 2014 vol. 82 no. 10 Supplement S12.007 (summary at http://www.neurology.org/content/82/10_Supplement/S12.007)

15. Connect - the communication difficulty network, in London SE1, information online at http://www.ukconnect.org

16. Jill Bolte Taylor. *My Stroke of Insight: a brain scientist's personal journey*, Hodder & Stoughton, 2008.

17. Robert McCrum. *My Year Off: Rediscovering Life After a Stroke*, Picador, 1998.

18. Tom Balchin. *The Successful Stroke Survivor*. Bagwin, 2011.

19. John Gillespie Magee. *High Flight*, 1941. The poem and other details of Magee's life are at https://en.wikipedia.org/wiki/John_Gillespie_Magee,_Jr.

20. MJ O'Donnell. Feet on the ground - being an approach to modern verse. Blackie, 1946.

21. Edith Sitwell. Still falls the rain (the raids 1940, night and dawn), 1940, in *The Penguin Poets: Edith Sitwell - a selection by the author, Penguin Books, 1952*.
    A recording of Edith Sitwell reading the poem is at http://www.poetryarchive.org/poem/still-falls-rain

22. Gerard Manley Hopkins. God's grandeur, in e.g. *The Illustrated Poets: Gerard Manley Hopkins*, Aurum Press, 1993.

23. Irina Ratushinskaya. *Pencil Letter*, Bloodaxe Books Ltd, 1988.

24. Jim Cotter. *Etched by Silence: a pilgrim engages with the poems and questions of RS Thomas*. DVD, Cairns Publications, 2013.

25. Hermione Lee. *Virginia Woolf*. Vintage, 1997.

26. Virginia Woolf. The Humane Art (1940) in *The Death of the Moth, and Other Essays*. Harcourt Publishers Ltd, 1974.

27. Elisabeth Schüssler Fiorenza. *Bread not Stone: the challenge of feminist Biblical interpretation*, T&T Clark, 1990.

28. Phyllis Trible. *Texts of terror: literary-feminist readings of Biblical narratives*, SCM Press, 1992.

29. Mark Haddon. *The Curious Incident of the Dog in the Night-time*, Vintage, 2004.

30. Karen Armstrong. *Through the Narrow Gate*, Flamingo, 1997; *Beginning the World*, Pan Books, 1984; *The Spiral Staircase*, Harper Perennial, 2005.

31. AE Housman. *A Shropshire Lad*, 1896. Section XL. Online at e.g. http://www.theotherpages.org/poems/housm03.html

32. Major sources of information and support include the Alzheimer's Society in the UK, at www.alzheimers.org.uk

33. Information about vascular dementia and contacts in various countries can be found at http://www.helpguide.org/articles/alzheimers-dementia/

vascular-dementia.htm and also http://www.bloodpressureuk.org/
BloodPressureandyou/Yourbody/Dementia

34. Admiral Nurses are part of Dementia UK; details (including the origin of
their name from one of their clients) are at www.dementiauk.org/about-us

35. A large international study from 2016 is: Blood Pressure and Risk of
Vascular Dementia - Evidence from a Primary Care Registry and a
Cohort Study of Transient Ischemic Attack and Stroke, authors CA
Emdin and colleagues. *Stroke* 2016;47:1429-1435 with an online
summary at http://stroke.ahajournals.org/content/47/6/1429

36. AE Housman. *A Shropshire Lad*, 1896. Section XLIII. Online at http://
www.theotherpages.org/poems/housm04.html

37. Sally Magnusson. *Where memories go: why dementia changes everything*,
Two Roads, 2014.

38. Keith Ward. *More than matter - what humans really are*, Lion Books,
2010, page 73.

39. Sandi Toksvig. *Whistling for the Elephants*. Sphere, 2002.

40. Mary Ann Shaffer and Annie Barrows. *The Guernsey Literary and Potato
Peel Pie Society*, Bloomsbury Publishing, 2010, page 7.

41. Katherine B Nuckolls, John Cassel, Berton H Kaplan. *Psychological assets,
life crisis and the prognosis of pregnancy*. American Journal of Epidemiology
95: 431-441, 1972. The abstract is online at http://aje.oxfordjournals.
org/content/95/5/431

42. Cary Cherniss. *Beyond Burnout: Helping Teachers, Nurses, Therapists and
Lawyers Recover from Stress and Disillusionment*, Routledge, 1995.

43. From Dylan Thomas's poem *Do not go gentle into that good night* from *In
Country Sleep, And Other Poems*, 1952.

44. The Rosetta Stone is said to be the most visited exhibit in the British
Museum in London, with parallel texts in Egyptian hieroglyphics,
Egyptian script, and Greek.

45. Stephen Mitchell. *The Book of Job*, North Point Press, 1987.

46. George Bernard Shaw. *The Doctor's Dilemma*. Penguin, 1946.

47. Thomas Hobbes. *Of Man, Being the First Part of Leviathan.* Chapter
XIII. Of the Natural Condition of Mankind as Concerning Their Felicity

and Misery, 1651. Available online at http://www.bartleby.com/34/5/13. html with the well-known quotation at the end of the ninth paragraph.

48. John Henry Newman. *The Dream of Gerontius*, 1865. The text is in the Sixth Phase, spoken by the Angel of the Agony (sung by the Angel in Part 2 of Elgar's setting, 1900).

49. In *Bacchae* by Euripides, about 400BCE.

50. Douglas Adams. *Life, the universe and everything*, Pan Books, 1982.

51. Elizabeth Barrett Browning. *To Flush my dog*, published 1844.

52. John Suchet. *My Bonnie – how dementia stole the love of my life*, Harper, 2011.

53. George Bernard Shaw. Maxim 124 in the section on Reason in *Maxims for Revolutionists*, 1903.

54. Mackellar D. *My Country*, first published 1908. Included in *The Wide Brown Land*, an anthology of Australian verse first published in 1934. As of May 2016 there is a video on YouTube of Dorothea Mackellar herself reading the full poem *My Country*, at https://www.youtube.com/watch?v=o5bNhQrKay0.

55. Peter Lanyon. From a biography at the Tate Gallery exhibition 2010-11. I have been unable to trace the source of the quotation. Also from the Courtauld Gallery exhibition 2016.

56. Simon Schama. *Landscape and Memory*, Harper Perennial, 2004.

57. Vincent van Gogh's painting *Wheatfield with Crows* is in the van Gogh Museum in Amsterdam, as is *Harvest with Blue Cart* and *Wheatfield with Lark*.

58. TS Eliot. The thoughts are the last lines of the poem *East Coker*, the second of the Four Quartets, from 1940. In e.g. *TS Eliot, Collected Poems 1909-1962*, Faber and Faber, 1974.

59. Vikram Seth. *An Equal Music*, 1999.

60. Nicholas Spice. Review of *An Equal Music* in London Review of Books, 29 April 1999.

61. William Harris. *Bring us O Lord* - anthem for double choir, 1959, on YouTube at https://www.youtube.com/watch?v=DogQazxXdYk

The words are a prayer by Eric Milner White, the central section of which is based on the final sentences of a long sermon preached by John Donne at Whitehall (London) on 29 February 1627-28. The full text of the sermon is accessible at, for example, http://www.biblestudytools. com/classics/the-works-of-john-donne-vol-5/sermon-cxlvi.html

62. The CD was of Angela Hewitt playing on the piano the first book of the Well-Tempered Clavier (the 48) by JS Bach.

63. Margaret Rizza's biography can be viewed at http://www.margaretrizza. com/biography.html which also refers to her music.

64. Sacred Music DVD: Series One COR16078. Commentary by Simon Russell Beale, music by The Sixteen with Harry Christophers. Series Two was shown on the BBC but there is no DVD.

65. Victoria, God's Composer DVD: COR16100. Commentary by Simon Russell Beale, music by The Sixteen with Harry Christophers.

66. Felix Mendelssohn. *Octet in E-flat major, opus 20*, 1825. On YouTube at www.youtube.com/watch?v=pY_gbooPwoc with the rising theme at the beginning of the first movement.

67. Robert Browning, *Andrea del Sarto*, in *Robert Browning: Men and Women and other poems*, Everyman (JM Dent & Charles E Tuttle) 1993. The poet writes as the artist in conversation with his model - his muse and lover. The poem ends on rather a different note, "I am grown peaceful as old age tonight," but still thinking about "heaven, perhaps new chances."

68. Strauss, Richard. *Beim Schlafengehen* from *Four Last Songs*, 1948. Words by Herman Hesse. On YouTube at www.youtube.com/ watch?v=Se0HPsJex04 sung by Jessye Norman; the rising theme is in the violin at 2 minutes and 30 seconds, and in the voice at 3 minutes and 40 seconds.

69. Frederic Chopin. *Scherzo No 2 in B flat minor, opus 31*, 1837. On YouTube at www.youtube.com/watch?v=S94Nh-bSomo played by Kristian Zimerman. The rising theme is at 4 minutes and 45 seconds, and at 6 minutes and 35 seconds.

70. William Byrd. Reasons briefly set down by the author, to persuade every one to learn to sing. In *Psalms, Sonnets and Songs*, 1588. The full list of reasons is accessible at, for example, http://www.ancientgroove.co.uk/ books/ByrdReasons.pdf

71. Johnny Cash singing *Daddy Sang Bass* can be viewed at https://www.youtube.com/watch?v=NGUP8oc9Bgs

72. Edward Elgar, *Sea Pictures, opus 37*, 1899. The recording which I first heard, sung by Janet Baker, is available on YouTube (at 12 May 2016) at https://www.youtube.com/watch?v=GauIMo8Manc

73. Anthony Storr. *Music and the Mind*, Harper Collins, 1997, page 7.

74. Hal Hodson. Talking gibbonish: deciphering the banter of the apes, *New Scientist*, 10 January 2015.

75. Margaret Rizza. An interview in *For a Change* magazine of April 1, 2003, at www.thefreelibrary.com under Humanities>Philosophy and Religion

76. Vladimir Ashkenazy in 1968, aged 30; in a Christopher Nupen film, shown on BBC4 in 2008.

77. Robert Schumann. *On Music and Musicians*, edited by Konrad Wollf, translated by Paul Rosenfeld, University of California Press, 1983, page 121.

78. Howard Goodall, at the beginning of episode 3 of Channel 4 TV series *How Music Works*, 2006. On YouTube at https://www.youtube.com/watch?v=KwRHu8T1lCs

79. Wolfgang Amadeus Mozart. *Concerto Rondo for piano and orchestra K382*, 1782. The first version I heard is available (May 2016) on YouTube at https://www.youtube.com/watch?v=t_tDfnYVHMY

80. Clive Sansom. *The Shepherds' Carol, in The Witnesses and Other Poems*, Methuen, 1956, page 104.

81. Aldous Huxley. *Music at Night*. Triad Grafton, 1986, page 20.

82. Sara Maitland. *A Book of Silence*. Granta Books, 2009. She discusses reading (pages 146 and following) amongst many aspects of silence.

83. Barry Morley. *Fire at the Center - a new look at Quaker religious education*. Baltimore Yearly Quaker Meeting, undated. The pdf document can be downloaded from http://www.bym-rsf.org/publications/overview.html where there is a link in the centre near the foot of the page.

84. Reported by James Breslin, *Mark Rothko: A Biography*. University of Chicago Press, 1998, page 539.

85. RS Thomas. *Kneeling*, in *RS Thomas Selected Poems 1946-1968*, Bloodaxe Books, 1986.

86. Vikram Seth, *An Equal Music*, 1999. The thought is on page 85 in the Phoenix paperback edition, 6th impression, 2000.

87. Thomas Cranmer added those words to earlier Latin texts in his English version of the marriage service published in the Book of Common Prayer of 1549.

88. Mary Warnock. *An Intelligent Person's Guide to Ethics*, Duckworth, 1998, page 89.

89. Mary Warnock. *Dishonest to God – on keeping religion out of politics*, Continuum, 2010, chapter 4 pages 112-3.

90. Sarah Coakley. *The Mathematics of Evolutionary Biology - Implications for Ethics, Teleology and 'Natural Theology'*. Gresham College Lecture, London, 3 February 2016. Online at http://www.gresham.ac.uk/lectures-and-events/the-mathematics-of-evolutionary-biology-implications-for-ethics

91. Martin A Nowak. Five Rules for the Evolution of Cooperation. *Science* 2006 Dec 8; 314(5805): 1560–1563. Also Martin Nowak with Roger Highfield: *Super Cooperators: Evolution, Altruism and Human Behaviour (Why We Need Each Other to Succeed)*, Canongate, 2011.

92. Hans Küng and Karl-Josef Kuschel, editors. *A Global Ethic: The Declaration of the Parliament of the World's Religions*, SCM Press, 1993, pages 14-15.

93. *A Global Ethic*, page 23.

94. Rodrigue Tremblay. *The Code for Global Ethics: 10 Humanist Principles*. Prometheus, 2010.

95. John Harris. *The Value of Life: An introduction to medical ethics*, Routledge, 1989.

96. Carol Gilligan. *In a Different Voice*, Harvard University Press, 1993, page 100. The other ideas from Gilligan are from pages xiv and 62.

97. Christine Gudorf, Parenting, mutual love and sacrifice, Chapter 12 in *Women's Consciousness, Women's Conscience: A Reader in Feminist Ethics*, Harper and Row, 1987, ed Andolsen, Gudorf, Pellauer, pages 182 and 185.

98. Raimond Gaita, *A Common Humanity: thinking about love and truth and justice*, Routledge, 2nd edition, 2000, page 19.

99. Andrew Miller. *Oxygen*, Sceptre, 2001, page 308

100. J Scott Peck. *The Road Less Travelled*, Hutchinson, 1983, page 81.

101. Charles Darwin. 'Our poor child, Annie', Note of reminiscence of Anne Elizabeth Darwin, 30 April 1851. Online at: http://darwin-online.org.uk/content/frameset?pageseq=1&item ID=CUL-DAR210.13.40&viewtype=text

102. Charles Darwin. Darwin Correspondence Project, Letter 4348. Darwin, CR to Hooker, JD, 27 November 1863. Online at: http://www.darwinproject.ac.uk/letter/DCP-LETT-4348.xml

103. Nick Lane. *Life Ascending: The Ten Great Inventions of Evolution*, Profile Books, 2009.

104. Samuel Beckett. *Waiting for Godot/En Attendant Godot*, Grove Press, 2010.

105. Samuel Beckett. *The Unnamable* in *Three Novels: Molloy, Malone Dies, the Unnamable*, Grove Press, 2009.

106. Clive James. *Sentenced to life - poems 2011-2014*, Picador, 2015. The poem is Rounded with a Sleep, page 44.

107. Terry Pratchett. *A Slip of the Keyboard*, Corgi, 2015. The quotation was from 2008.

108. The music specially composed by Ane Brun for the final episode of the Swedish version of Wallander (with Krister Henriksson in the title role) is on YouTube at https://www.youtube.com/watch?v=UGssssSZUKI (accessed in June 2016)

109. Henning Mankel, *The Troubled Man: A Kurt Wallander Mystery*. Vintage, 2012, page 30.

110. Mary Shelley, *The Last Man*, 1826. This is a science fiction novel later than Frankenstein. In Volume 3 chapter 2 one of her female characters says, ".. the true love I bear you will render this and every other loss endurable." The text can also be viewed at http://www.freeclassicebooks.com/Shelley%20Mary/The%20Last%20Man.pdf with the quotation on page 445.

111. CG Jung, *Memories, Dreams, Reflections.* Vintage Books, 1965. The quotation is from near the end of section I of chapter XII, Late Thoughts. With the preceding sentence it reads, "Meaninglessness inhibits fullness of life and is therefore equivalent to illness. Meaning makes a great many things endurable perhaps everything." The scanned full text of the book is accessible at e.g. https://archive.org/stream/MemoriesDreamsReflectionsCarlJung/Memories,%20Dreams,%20Reflections%20-%20Carl%20Jung_djvu.txt